ADVANCE PRAISE

That an ounce of prevention is worth several pounds of cure is especially true for the brain. As Dr. Michael Lewis points out in this seminal book, if you don't have sufficient levels of omega-3 fatty acids in the brain, you are at great potential risk for future neurological problems. When such events do occur, especially with severe brain trauma, you will require very high-dose interventions of omega-3 fatty acids to resolve the condition. When Brains Collide is an extremely valuable asset for anyone with a loved one whose life is being compromised by ongoing brain trauma.

— Barry Sears, PhD, Leading Research Scientist and author of number-one New York Times best seller *The Zone*

Michael Lewis has taken an understanding of the new evidence of omega-3s on brain cell structures, signalling, and for the resolution of inflammation to a new dimension of addressing serious brain trauma.

If the brain is damaged—just like damage to any building or machine—you need the right materials for restoration. The difficulty with the brain is twofold: First, it takes a short time for serious damage to result in inflammation, brain cell death, and scarring with permanent disability. Secondly, we do not have the right building units to offer for repair.

Michael's approach of fast, instant treatment, and high dose levels of omega-3s is logical and evidence-based. Serious brain trauma cannot be dealt with by a randomised controlled trial. His approach, which has demonstrated some remarkable successes, needs serious consideration, especially when trauma can otherwise lead to grave disability.

— Michael A. Crawford, PhD, FRSB, FRCPath; Faculty of Medicine, Imperial College, London; Author of *Nutrition and Evolution: Food in Evolution and the Future*

The recipe for a good medical read has three main ingredients: it must be based on science, include personal experience, and have a sprinkle of common sense. Neuroscientist Dr. Michael Lewis compiles his decades of research and healing testimonies into a brain-health plan that works. This book gives hope to readers, especially persons suffering a traumatic brain injury, as well as a plan for how to heal.

The Omega-3 Protocol in this book puts to work the most important brain-healing medicine: omega-3 fats. Along with the thousands of medical journal articles proving the healing effects of omega-3s, Dr. Lewis's protocol partners science with common sense. The brain is mostly comprised of fat. Yes, we are "fatheads." Omega-3 fats are the most important building blocks of brain tissue. Therefore, it makes sense that omega-3s, in the healthful doses recommended in this book, help an injured brain to heal.

– William Sears, MD, Author, *The Omega-3 Effect* and more than forty other best-selling books

In his book When Brains Collide, Dr. Michael Lewis provides a well-tested format on how to improve the way we address prevention and treatment of all forms of traumatic brain injury. The West Point grad and retired Army Colonel is a nationally recognized authority in the treatment of traumatic brain injuries and has developed The Omega-3 Protocol for dealing with the devastating effects, at times, of the postconcussion syndrome. His description of the neuro-protective, anti-inflammatory, and neuro-regenerative properties of essential fatty acids (fish oil!) provides the basis for fish oil being the number-one consumed supplement in the United States. This book is concise, complete, and filled with personal success stories that can be appreciated by all.

– Joseph C. Maroon, MD, author and Clinical Professor Neurosurgery, University of Pittsburgh; Team Neurosurgeon, The Pittsburgh Steelers

I applaud Michael Lewis's groundbreaking work. It is a lifesaver that has impacted my life both personally and professionally as The Sneaky Chef, and as a mom on a mission committed to children's health.

– Missy Chase Lapine, creator of the wildly successful *Sneaky Chef* series of books, including New York Times best seller *The Sneaky Chef: Simple Strategies for Hiding Healthy Foods in Kids' Favorite Meals.*

Dr. Lewis has revealed himself to be a great storyteller in relating a major contemporary issue of society. He clearly highlights the influence of traumatic brain injury (TBI) as going beyond the medical implications. We now know that TBI also impacts greater health-care issues and the well-being of patients through its potential long-term consequences, since it is the number-one environmental cause of dementias such as Alzheimer's disease.

Dr. Lewis touches upon how using omega-3 fatty acids, as part of therapeutic approaches to combat these conditions, can potentially offer breakthroughs in slowing down or reversing the consequences of TBI. This book builds upon the premise that there is a need for a better understanding of TBI so that new, effective therapeutic approaches can be developed to defeat this condition.
    – Nicolas G. Bazan, MD, PhD; Founder and Director, Neuroscience
        Center of Excellence, LSU Health New Orleans

The use of omega-3 fatty acids for treatment of brain injury and disorders is an emerging field now with innumerable published studies and medical science support. Dr. Mike Lewis has been an innovator in omega-3 use, and he details his experience and that of his patients in When Brains Collide. The stories and plight of his patients, as well as the journey of discovery of a new form of dietary supplement support for the brain at a time when there is no comparable pharmaceutical answer, are fascinating and should spur others to action.
    – Julian Bailes, MD, FACS; Chairman, Department of
        Neurosurgery and Co-Director, NorthShore Neurological
        Institute, Chicago; Medical Director, Center for Study of
        Retired Athletes, University of North Carolina, Chapel Hill

This book reflects the passion, energy, and dedication Dr. Michael Lewis has given to one of the most challenging questions in medicine: how to improve recovery after injury of the brain. This remains an area where there is a need for much progress and therapeutic innovation. Dr. Lewis explains the complexity of the events that follow a brain injury and highlights how the present management of this often life-changing condition is very limited even in developed countries. The book explores in depth the potential of omega-3 fatty acids, natural compounds whose remarkable properties have been much researched in the last decade. Dr. Lewis adopts a pragmatic approach and gives examples of several case histories from his own practice, which support the concept that omega-3 fatty acids have significant neuro-protective and neuro-regenerative potential.

Through his Brain Health Education and Research Institute and the present book, Dr. Lewis shows an exemplary focus of purpose to change attitudes and accept nonconventional solutions that benefit patients, and thus he also offers a new perspective on the specific nutritional and metabolic support required after neurotrauma—a chapter yet to be written in modern medicine.

Brain injury is often the first step leading to a delayed neurodegenerative process. The thoughts articulated in this book, on the importance of safe prophylaxis and also prompt intervention, whether in a civilian or military context, should encourage much reflection on a new way of approaching the management of brain injury in the twenty-first century.

> – Adina Michael-Titus, MSc, DSc.; Professor of Neuroscience, Centre for Neuroscience and Trauma, Barts and The London School of Medicine and Dentistry

Finally, medical news everyone can use. Colonel Michael Lewis, MD, doctor to generals and policy makers, explains with personal stories and down-to-earth language successes of omega-3 DHA in aiding recovery after traumatic brain injury. A notable book every brain should read.

> – Tom Brenna, PhD; Professor of Human Nutrition, Cornell University; President, International Society for the Study of Fatty Acids and Lipids

Dr. Michael Lewis is an omega-3 maverick. He clearly knows the potential benefits of fish oils in cases of traumatic brain injury, and reports them. If only the traditional medical community would just listen instead of saying no!

> – Mark L. Gordon, MD; Interventional Endocrinologist and Director, The Millennium Health Centers, Inc.; Medical Director, Millennium-Warrior Angels Foundation TBI Project

Brain injury survivors, caregivers, and professionals will find in these pages an innovative, safe, affordable, and practical approach to "fighting the brain injury wars," offering realistic hope against what are often intractable challenges.

Twelve years after our teenage son suffered a severe brain injury in a car accident, we discovered Dr. Lewis's Omega-3 Protocol. Bart made dramatic gains in short-term memory, executive function, and fine motor control. After more than a decade's hiatus, once again he is right-side dominant—eating, writing, even playing guitar as a righty. There is practically no precedent for such recovery so long postinjury. Our family remains astounded, delighted, and ever so grateful to Dr. Lewis.

— Joel Goldstein, author of *No Stone Unturned: A Father's Memoir of His Son's Encounter with Traumatic Brain Injury*, and Executive Director of the BART Foundation

Dr. Michael Lewis has worked tirelessly to bridge the gap between military medicine and the natural wellness revolution. He possesses the values, skill, and leadership that our failing medical system desperately needs today. Learn how Dr. Lewis invented a new, safe, and effective way to support the body's innate healing process from traumatic brain injury, using natural remedies and noninvasive imaging. This book will give you the power to heal, the power to change, and the confidence to know that one of America's greatest physicians hears you."

— Stuart Tomc, VP of Human Nutrition, CV Sciences, Inc.

Dr. Lewis provides a uniquely compelling argument for omega-3 supplementation, particularly in high doses for those who are suffering from traumatic brain injury. Importantly, this book inspires a call to action for transformative, efficacious therapeutic interventions to address the national concussion epidemic.

— Michael E. Singer, PhD; Chief Executive Officer, BrainScope Company, Inc.; Former President of Revolution Health Investments

Dr. Lewis has written a compelling book, giving new hope to those who suffer the lingering effects of traumatic brain injury (TBI) and their loved ones. When Brains Collide skillfully combines the latest scientific research with interesting stories of those living with TBI and their experiences applying The Omega-3 Protocol for concussion.

— Steve Dubin, Principal, SDA Ventures LLC; Former CEO, Martek Biosciences, Inc.

Prior to my son Grant's accident, I had no idea how common traumatic brain injuries (TBIs) were. I also had no idea how much can be done for them. Now that I know both of these things, I am determined to be part of the solution and to help support those who are out on the front lines making a difference. Dr. Michael Lewis is one of our big heroes in brain injury research and one of the reasons Grant is thriving today.

I hope you will share this book and his fantastic blog with everyone you know. We are all touched by TBIs, and there is so much that we can do. There are so many lives and brains that can be saved by this information.
— JJ Virgin, New York Times best-selling author, prominent fitness and nutrition expert, public speaker and media personality

Our son Bobby was in a very serious car accident that left him with a traumatic brain injury and in coma for more than two months. Doctors gave us no hope of his staying alive, let alone coming out of his coma. When we heard about omega-3s and Dr. Lewis's research, we decided to take on the hospital and the doctors to allow our son to have the omega-3s ASAP. It was a very difficult battle, but they finally agreed. We strongly believe that it was the omega-3s that accelerated his recovery and shortened all our suffering.

Bobby is still taking high doses of fish oil and is a strong advocate for the omega-3s that help his depression and anxiety. He has improved from two years of wheelchair and two years of walker to now using only a cane. We are grateful that Dr. Mike Lewis has supported us from Bobby's first days in the hospital six years ago and still to this day. That is the kind of doctor he is. He has been available to us any day or night or weekend. He is family to us because he cares deeply for us and loves Bobby as much as we love him.
— Peter Ghassemi, father of Bobby, a severe traumatic brain injury victim featured on CNN's Sanjay Gupta, MD, show

I have been fortunate to work with Dr. Lewis and some of his patients, including Bobby, to see firsthand how high-dose fish oil can be life changing. Even with my own son, I have found comfort in knowing that he can take fish oil preventively during football season to help nourish and protect his brain. Dr. Lewis has helped bring important awareness to brain health and sport concussion that is invaluable and ahead of its time!
— Keri Marshall, ND; Director, Global Lipid Science and Advocacy, Royal DSM N.V.; Former Chief Medical Officer, Nordic Naturals, Inc.

Dr. Lewis is a pioneer in the treatment and management of brain injuries with diet and lifestyle. He is a unique example of taking cutting-edge basic and animal research and translating it into clinical practice under the most dire circumstances. I was first introduced to his work when trying to help our soldiers manage the trauma of combat, and I have only grown to respect him more since. He has taken the theory of saturating the brain with the nutrients it is comprised of in response to injuries to real-life settings and has seen some stunning success stories. As more clinical science develops in this area, I know Michael will be integral in guiding its practical use.

– Adam Ismail, Executive Director, Global Organization for EPA and DHA Omega-3s

Mike Lewis is a founding member of the Pop Warner Medical Advisory Committee, helping to keep us at the forefront of player health and safety. Consisting of approximately 325,000 young people ranging from ages five to sixteen years old, Pop Warner is the largest youth football, cheer, and dance program in the world. When Brains Collide is just one example of the knowledge and experience Dr. Lewis lends to us. We deeply value his input, feedback, and generosity with his time and efforts on behalf of all the young scholar-athletes in Pop Warner Football and Cheer.

– Jon Butler, Executive Director, Pop Warner Little Scholars Football and Cheer

Dr. Mike Lewis is one of the thought-leading experts in our country on concussions and traumatic brain injuries (TBIs). We have recommended his approach and the importance of omega-3s/fish oil for many years in our integrative pharmacy, Village Green Apothecary. His protocol has made tremendous positive impacts in the speed of recovery for our clients.

The impact of concussions and TBIs is at an all-time high. If you, a family member, or a friend has been impacted by a concussion or a TBI, you should start by reading Dr. Lewis's book—this is game-changing information!

– Marc Isaacson, CEO, Village Green Apothecary/IQYou

Dr. Mike Lewis makes a very strong case that omega-3 fatty acids found in the marine environment have great potential for protecting the brain from life-altering outcomes due to traumatic brain injury, and for aiding in its healing after such an injury. The preclinical (basic science) evidence is strong in this regard, and more research in which omega-3s are investigated in humans for improving clinical outcomes is clearly warranted. My own research has not been in the field of omega-3 fatty acid protective benefits prior to or after a traumatic brain injury. However, I have shown that these fatty acids modulate aspirin's effects on platelet function and inflammation in humans. Since they are safe, inexpensive, and without concerning interactions with drugs, their use should be more widespread, particularly in those whose information is studied carefully after a traumatic brain injury. The brain is a very malleable organ, and let's take advantage of this!

– Robert C. Block, MD, MPH, FACP, FNLA; Associate
Professor of Cardiology and Public Health Sciences,
University of Rochester Medical Center

I extend my deep gratitude to Dr. Lewis and others working so hard to get this important information out to the millions of people it can help. Considering how common traumatic brain injuries (TBIs) are, there's a very good chance that one day you or someone close to you will be touched by TBI. Please read this important book and share it with others. The life you save may be your own.

– Randy Hartnell, President & CEO, Vital Choice
Wild Seafood & Organics, VitalChoice.com

WHEN BRAINS COLLIDE

WHEN
BRAINS
COLLIDE

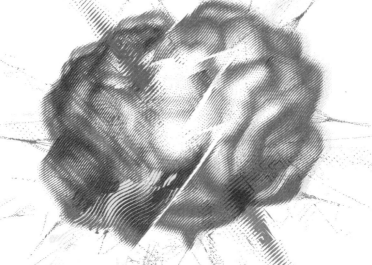

WHAT EVERY ATHLETE AND PARENT SHOULD KNOW
ABOUT THE PREVENTION AND TREATMENT
OF CONCUSSIONS AND HEAD INJURIES

MICHAEL D. LEWIS, MD
FOREWORD BY JJ VIRGIN

DISCLAIMER

The information provided in this book is designed to provide helpful information on the subjects discussed. This book is not meant to be used, nor should it be used, to diagnose or treat any medical condition. For diagnosis or treatment of any medical problem, consult your own physician. The publisher and author are not responsible for any specific health or allergy needs that may require medical supervision and are not liable for any damages or negative consequences from any treatment, action, application or preparation, to any person reading or following the information in this book. References are provided for informational purposes only and do not constitute endorsement of any products, websites, or other sources. Readers should be aware that the websites listed in this book may change.

WHEN BRAINS COLLIDE

What Every Athlete and Parent Should Know
about the Prevention and Treatment of
Concussions and TBI

ISBN   978-1-61961-492-5 *Paperback*

978-1-61961-493-2 *Ebook*

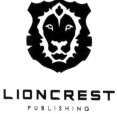

LIONCREST
PUBLISHING

This book is dedicated to my fellow military veterans, many of whom have sacrificed and continue to sacrifice much for their country. My hope is that this book provides a way forward for you.

CONTENTS

FOREWORD

BY JJ VIRGIN

"Now we wait," said Grant's doctor.

"We wait?" I asked. "Surely there must be something we can do to speed the healing process?"

"Nope, not a thing. Now it is up to time."

Thankfully, I am not known for my patience. It would not have served my sixteen-year old son, who was slowly emerging from a two-week coma with a severe traumatic brain injury (TBI) along with thirteen fractures and a torn aorta.

The local hospital's head trauma doctor advised us to let our son go, but we overruled him and had him air-lifted to Harbor UCLA where Dr. Carlos Donayre repaired Grant's torn aorta. A torn aorta kills 90 percent of accident victims at the scene. Without surgery, it would have ruptured completely and killed him within twenty-four hours.

Once he was out of this immediate danger, I tapped into my extensive network of health professionals to figure out the best next steps for Grant's neurological condition. The victim of a hit-and-run driver while out walking in our neighborhood at dusk, my son was now just supposed to give his recovery over to time.

I kept hearing about high-dose fish oil: how it was used to help Randal McCloy, the sole survivor from the Sago Mine accident in January 2006 in West Virginia, and how it also helped a kid not much older than Grant, who was in a severe car accident in northern Virginia. Someone pointed Grant's father, John, to CNN.com and a special segment on the Sanjay Gupta, MD, show that detailed how these two cases were related.

John reached out to Sanjay Gupta and his producer, Stephanie Smith, who contacted Drs. Michael Lewis and Julian Bailes, the two physicians featured on Sanjay's show. Coincidently, I had met Mike Lewis earlier that year at a conference in Orlando. Dr. Lewis immediately responded to John, explaining the doses and the protocol for using omega-3s for severe brain injury. I also was fortunate to have Dr. Barry Sears send me the research behind why they used omega-3s for Randal McCloy.

Facts help. I was already a big believer and user of fish oil. Grant was on 5 grams of fish oil at the time of the accident, which I believe played a critical role in protecting his brain in the first place. I was convinced that this was one of the key therapeutic interventions I wanted for Grant. The challenge was convincing the hospital. Grant had multiple brain bleeds along with severe road rash, multiple fractures, lacerated kidneys, and severe bruising. The doctors were concerned that adding fish oil would create bleeding problems. I shared all of the research from Dr. Sears, which clearly showed that fish oil does not increase bleed times, but they wouldn't budge. They were only willing to give him 2 grams of fish oil through his feeding tube.

I knew from all of the research and the experts I was consulting with that there was no risk to Grant to increase his fish oil, so as soon as Grant managed to get rid of his feeding tube (he actually coughed it out himself), we started increasing his fish oil dose ourselves. I did this whenever I knew they were going to run labs to access his bleeding time to ensure that bleeding wasn't an issue. I was literally sneaking it in when the nurses left the room, bringing it in every day in a cooler bag so it would be fresh. At that first hospital, I managed to get him up to 5 to 10 grams a day.

Then we had him moved to Children's Hospital of LA (CHLA) as he improved and became ready to begin rehabilitation. When I arrived, I told the medical team that he was on 20 grams of fish oil, so they just wrote that into his daily dosage of medicines. The shift to 20 grams of fish oil, as recommended by Dr. Lewis, was dramatic. When we were at Harbor UCLA, Grant's speech was fairly limited to "yes," "no," and "let's go." A day after we started him on the higher dose, he called me on his iPhone in the middle of the night and we had a conversation. I woke up the next morning and assumed I had dreamed the whole thing until a nurse confirmed the call!

From that point forward, things moved fairly quickly. When we arrived at CHLA, Grant didn't know who he was, sometimes he didn't know who I was, and he could barely feed himself. He had to relearn everything—how to walk, draw, brush his teeth, and so on. It was like raising a very big baby very quickly.

Grant came home five months after the accident. The team at CHLA wanted us to stay longer, but we felt Grant needed to be around his family and home and that we could design a rehabilitation program near home. This was definitely more difficult, but I believe it has been better for Grant.

The biggest challenge with all of this was the lack of support and resources. When I came home and started looking for what we could put together for Grant, I was amazed at how little was available. We put together a fantastic team and services to support Grant in his recovery including hyperbaric oxygen therapy, SPECT scan monitoring with Dr. Daniel Amen of the Amen Clinic, neurofeedback, exercise, speech therapy, and art therapy. And of course, I modified aspects of his diet and supplementation to support healing and help reduce inflammation.

This has all helped Grant improve, but he's been isolated. I have been frustrated by the lack of support for TBI sufferers. Grant missed his junior year of high school and has never been able to get back to high school. His friends didn't know how to deal with him. Coming out of a brain injury is very akin to going on a roller-coaster ride and not knowing when it will end. Over the first year, he would get angry, impatient, and frustrated. He didn't know how to relate to others anymore, and high school kids are not exactly patient and empathetic. I know there are others out there who are suffering, too, and we need a way to connect with one another.

In terms of using fish oil as treatment for TBI, I also realize how lucky Grant, Bobby Ghassemi, Randal McCloy, and the fortunate others like them are to have been able to use this treatment, because much of this information is not yet readily available or commonly being used in medical facilities. As I said, I had to go behind the backs of the medical team of Harbor UCLA despite having the research to support high-dose fish oil. I also brought meals, shakes, and supplements into the hospital and took control of Grant's nutrition.

It's been nearly four years since Grant's accident. In some ways he is doing better than before the accident—he is super creative, very empathetic, and confident. He has grown very interested in botany and has built a hydroponic garden in our backyard. He struggles with memory and has hearing loss in one ear. Modern technology makes these issues fairly easy to deal with, and he finds it can be convenient at times to be able to dial down his hearing aid and tune us all out! He will always be dealing with the ramifications of his TBI, but we've all learned that there is so much he can do for it.

Prior to Grant's accident, I had no idea how common TBIs were. I also had no idea how much can be done for them. Now that I know both of these things, I am determined to be part of the solution and to help support those who are out on the front lines making a difference. Dr. Michael Lewis is one of our big heroes in brain injury research and one of the reasons Grant is thriving today.

I hope you will share this book and his fantastic blog with everyone you know. We are all touched by TBIs, and there is so much that we can do. There are so many lives and brains that can be saved by this information.

– JJ VIRGIN
New York Times best-selling author, prominent fitness and nutrition expert, public speaker and media personality

INTRODUCTION

I was on the steps of the United States Capitol building in full dress uniform. It was Brain Injury Awareness Day at Congress, March 17, 2010, and the morning was sunny, a light breeze tossed leaves, and I was preoccupied with preparing for a series of meetings on traumatic brain injury (TBI). My phone vibrated in my pocket. A friend, who worked for the Food and Drug Administration (FDA) and served with me on the US Department of Defense Dietary Supplement Committee, seemed agitated on the other end. "Hey, this is Jerry. I need to ask you something."

My first thought was the FDA was questioning my recommendations to use omega-3 fatty acids in a nutritional approach for mild and severe head injuries. But as Jerry continued, it was clear this wasn't about committee work or the FDA.

"This is personal," he explained. "A friend of mine's

son was in a car accident a couple of days ago and was severely injured and has a severe traumatic brain injury. They don't expect him to live." I interrupted him because I had heard about this accident from another friend who also was close to that family. "How can I help, Jerry? I heard it was a horrible accident." He responded, "Would you talk to the father about the idea of maybe using fish oil like they did for the Sago Mine survivor?"

I thought for a moment. In the Sago Mine accident, fish oil, filled with omega-3s, had been used successfully for carbon monoxide poisoning, but it had never been used for a severe traumatic brain injury. It made sense that omega-3s should help, at least that's what I thought. It was why I was standing on those steps. I made a swift decision and told him, "If the father calls, I'd be happy to talk to him about the possibility."

Within minutes the phone vibrated again. This time it was Peter, the father. He was distraught and trying to figure out what he and his wife, as parents, could do for their son, Bobby. He asked me about the idea of administering massive doses of fish oil. He had heard from Jerry that this technique was used in 2006 for the sole survivor of the Sago Mine disaster. Peter understood fish oil had never been tried as a treatment for a devastating brain injury. But he was fighting for his only son and he would do anything for him. He needed specifics and wanted to know what kind of fish oil to buy, how much to give, how often, and how to convince the medical doctors treating Bobby to move forward with this nutritional plan.

I thought fast. I knew there was a Whole Foods nearby just down the street from the Inova Fairfax Hospital where Bobby lay in a coma fighting for his life. I told Peter to look for liquid concentrated fish oil. He asked me what kind. My answer must have sounded generic, but it was the truth. "I don't know, anything. Just buy a liquid concentrate and start pouring it down his feeding tube. I think Nordic Naturals is a good brand, and they should have it at Whole Foods."

"How much?"

"Let's start with a tablespoon twice a day and we'll figure it out from there." I snapped the phone shut, after the mutual promise we would stay in touch.

The next day, I was at the National Institutes of Health (NIH) with a collaborator. We were finishing up a study that connected low omega-3 levels to increased risk of suicide in active-duty military. My phone rang again and this time it was the neurosurgeon treating Bobby. She explained that at the time of the accident he had suffered a subdural bleed. They had to surgically evacuate the blood pooling on his brain immediately following the accident. Then they had placed a monitor inside his skull to record the intracranial pressure and they put in a shunt to continue to drain his brain of accumulating fluid. In short, they had performed all the invasive techniques critical in acute neurosurgical care, and now here was Peter throwing a tantrum in the middle of the intensive care unit (ICU) insisting that his son start receiving high doses of fish oil.

Her questions rang with disbelief. "What are you doing? What are you trying to get us to do?"

"I believe the omega-3s in the fish oil will help with Bobby's recovery."

She paused. "We don't think he's going to survive. And it's been ten days since the accident. There is no reason to think anything will help at this point."

In the minutes that followed, we agreed there was no reason not to try.

That day, under the neurosurgeon's direction, the medical team began administering 15 milliliters of fish oil per day, saturating Bobby's brain with omega-3 fatty acids. That day also began Bobby's long road home.

Within two weeks, Bobby recovered enough to receive a tracheostomy to help with breathing and he was transported to Johns Hopkins University, Kennedy Krieger Hospital, for rehabilitation. Bobby's parents ensured that he continued to receive high doses of fish oil from the medical team at that facility. Three months later, against all odds, Bobby attended his high school graduation. Now, six years after his accident and concussion, Bobby still must face the challenges inherent with some physical disability, but he's a full-time college student working two part-time jobs. The omega-3s allowed his brain the chance to heal and he became the first patient suffering from a severe TBI to be treated specifically with high doses of fish oil.

The omega-3 fish oil protocol for severe TBI, though seemingly miraculous, was not developed in a vacuum. On January 2, 2006, fourteen miners were trapped in the Sago Mine in Upshur County, West Virginia. A methane gas explosion created a cave-in two miles below the surface, and though the fourteen men were trapped alive, it took forty-one hours to reach them. Tragically, by then only one man survived; the rest had succumbed to carbon monoxide poisoning. Randal L. McCloy Jr., was barely alive. Only twenty-six years old, he had suffered kidney, lung, liver, and heart damage, and lay in a coma.

When they pulled McCloy from the mine, the medical team started all the interventions required to treat carbon monoxide and methane gas poisoning. Hyperbaric oxygen was administered in an attempt to try to drive out the carbon monoxide and replace it with oxygen. Dialysis was used to reverse kidney failure. McCloy had suffered a massive heart attack and an anoxic brain injury, which meant there was no oxygen to his brain. As a result, he was left with very little brain function. Despite the terrible events, McCloy was, in a sense, lucky. His neurosurgeon was Dr. Julian Bailes.

Julian Bailes, MD, was the head of neurosurgery at

West Virginia University and friends with Dr. Barry Sears of the Zone Diet. Dr. Sears had been touting the anti-inflammatory benefits of omega-3s and when Bailes reached out to him, Sears agreed to help with treatment. They started pouring fish oil down McCloy's feeding tube to the point that the ICU smelled like a fish factory. Smell or no smell, McCloy's brain was saturated with omega-3 fatty acids.

Randy McCloy walked out of the hospital several months later and has gone on to father six children. He lives a relatively normal life with his wife of almost two decades. He has had as much as a full recovery as anybody could anticipate, and his recovery is actually quite remarkable. A few months later, as the press caught wind of the story and McCloy's remarkable recovery, Julian Bailes began the speaker circuit, explaining how omega-3s helped McCloy's brain to heal.

At the time, I was stationed in Bethesda at the Uniformed Services University of the Health Sciences, the military's medical school on the grounds of the National Naval Medical Center (it is now the Walter Reed National Military Medical Center). Though I was the head of Epidemiology and Biostatistics and focused on infectious diseases, I was constantly around men and women returning from Afghanistan and Iraq suffering from war injuries. There wasn't a time when I'd go to the gym and there wasn't a young soldier or Marine missing at least one limb, if not two or three, who was working out lifting weights, playing racquetball or basketball, or running on a treadmill. One time I found myself sharing the locker room with a soldier missing both legs from the waist down, lying on a bench struggling to get his gym clothes on. I offered to help but was quickly rebuffed with: "No, no, I got this." Men working out with one arm or leg missing, maybe both, or men and women with terrible burns and scar tissue is part of life on a military base. Seeing a guy running outside on two blades in place of his lower limbs is a regular occurrence.

One day later that same year, I was at a friend's house at Fort Myer to celebrate the Fourth of July. I'd known Jimmy and Maria McConville since we shared a house as junior officers when Jimmy and I served in the Cavalry together at Fort Ord, California. Now Jimmy was a two-star general (he subsequently earned a third star). We were outside in his backyard with a couple of other guys from our Cav days, nursing beers, and he leaned over, poked me in the chest, and said, "Mike, you're a doc. Why is Army research focused on trying to find a vaccine for malaria thirty years from now? We're at war. Help these guys. What are you doing about traumatic brain injury?"

And that became my driving question. What could I do to help? Watching a loved one suffer through a coma with severe brain trauma is like watching a slow-motion horror film unfold. Patients and their families are told by doctors and our medical system that there is nothing they can do. "Only time can heal the brain," they are told. The more I thought about that over the next few months, the more I refused to accept that premise. There must be something that can help our fellow soldiers recover better from TBI.

That year I continued to hear more and more about the Sago Mine disaster and how high doses of fish oil may have helped Randy McCloy. One evening, I was discussing this with a friend when he surprised me. "I know Julian Bailes—you want to talk to him?" He dialed his phone and handed it to me. I started peppering Dr. Bailes with question after question—why did he do this, and why did he do that? At one point he stopped me and said something about pouring fish oil down McCloy's feeding tube. I asked why he didn't give it intravenously since it would increase the blood levels very quickly. He said he didn't think an intravenous form of fish oil existed. (This gave me an idea, and I went on to invent an intravenous product high in omega-3s that is currently being tested by the Army and its industry partner).

With that conversation on my mind, the next day I went to the head of research for the Defense and Veterans Brain Injury Center located at Walter Reed Army Medical Center and asked, "Is anybody looking at the use of omega-3 fatty acids to help soldiers recover from traumatic brain injury?"

The director was very thoughtful, looked at me, and said, "No, why don't you?"

At this point in my professional career, I had served in the Army almost thirty years. My long history in the US Army began in my teens. Fresh from high school, I enrolled at the US Military Academy at West Point. I graduated and was commissioned as a Second Lieutenant in Military Intelligence. After graduating from Airborne and Ranger schools, I served in infantry divisions on the demilitarized zone in Korea and in California. When you've served your five-year commitment from West Point, you can leave the Army. But I decided at that point to go back to school. At West Point, my academic concentration was in Math, Chemistry, and Physics, with a minor in Civil Engineering. It was enough to get me the prerequisites for medical school. I had always wanted to be a doctor and really wanted to be a surgeon like my father. Four years later, I graduated from Tulane Medical School in New Orleans.

When I graduated, I did a surgical internship at Walter Reed Army Medical Center in Washington, DC. Back then, if you wanted to specialize, the Army would send you into general practice for a few years. The head of urologic surgery, which is the specialty I was planning to go into, arranged for me to be assigned to the Pentagon so that I'd be close by. I could come back to the hospital every week and do a half day of clinics in urology to keep my hand in it, so that when I started the residency, I'd pick up where I left off. I ended up spending four years at the Pentagon and went to aviation school to become a flight surgeon. I was the senior doctor in the group of general practitioners, so I was in charge of the primary-care and flight-medicine clinics at the Pentagon for a couple of years. As such, I was responsible for taking care of the 4-star Generals, the Chief of Staff and the Vice Chief of Staff of the Army, and the Secretary of the Army and their staff members, and my secretary handled all the active-duty and retired general officers who needed medical care. One of my retired general officers was the Chief Clerk of the Supreme Court, others were former Chairmen of the Joint Chiefs, and others were four-star generals, admirals, and dignitaries.

I also got to travel, a lot. One summer I volunteered on an interesting mission to Russia for a month, but that's a story for another time. I traveled with Congress all over the world, saw some amazing places and things, met leaders from around the world, and worked closely with Congressmen and Senators, keeping them healthy while traveling to some interesting corners of the world. It was a wonderful experience and I discovered that nights and weekends existed beyond marks on a calendar, something surgeons don't often get to experience.

When it became my time to go back to Walter Reed for surgical training, I decided instead to go into Preventive Medicine and Public Health, which took me to Johns Hopkins and then Walter Reed Army Institute of Research. When I was at Walter Reed Army Institute of Research, I invented and developed a novel bioterrorism warning system that was basically a massive data-mining system. All the Department of Defense's (DoD) health data was categorized and analyzed to determine if there was anything abnormal that might indicate the potential of a bioterrorism outbreak. This was in 1999.

The infectious diseases alert system I designed was titled "ESSENCE." It was essentially an anthrax warning system designed and implemented before anybody ever heard of anthrax and bioterrorism. The system I built and implemented is still running today. ESSENCE ultimately became an entire new branch of epidemiology focused on syndromic surveillance and stakeholders formed an international society. The program is in its sixteenth year and is used by every Health Department in the United States and is also used in many countries around the world.

My reward for designing and implementing ESSENCE was the freedom to explore whatever assignment I wanted. I chose to go to Bangkok, Thailand, to a special facility. The reason I wanted to go into Preventive Medicine was a new program started by the DoD called the Global Emerging Infections System, or GEIS for short. The Armed Forces Research Institute of Medical Sciences (AFRIMS) is a joint US Army/Royal Thai Army research lab in Bangkok established in 1958. AFRIMS is the premier research institute in all of Asia. I was asked to develop the GEIS program at AFRIMS to take advantage of this world-class asset. It was a two-year assignment where my job was to explore Asia looking for new and interesting diseases and develop partners to create programs like I had with ESSENCE. I was there when the SARS and Bird Flu outbreaks occurred, and I investigated some other fascinating disease outbreaks in the jungles of Nepal and the island nation of the Maldives. When 9/11 occurred, I was leading a multinational conference on disease surveillance in the foothills of Mount Everest in Nepal. Of course, immediately our military went to war in Afghanistan and Iraq while I continued to hunt diseases around Asia. Four years later, I was told I had valuable experience and was ordered to Bethesda to teach epidemiology to the medical students at the Military Medical School. It was there I began my interaction with wounded warriors and patients with traumatic brain injury.

All great solutions start with great questions, and that one question from the director of research served as mine. When I was asked, "Why don't you put together a study and figure it out?" I realized this was an extension of what I had been doing my whole career: think of an idea, ask a question, and design research to find an answer. I started to put together a research study at Walter Reed Army Medical Center and networked with top doctors, neurologists, and nutritionists just to identify who knew what about omega-3s and their function in the brain. It turned out that the number of individuals who have actually studied omega-3s in the brain is relatively small and those who knew anything about omega-3s and TBI was almost nonexistent. While I networked and learned as quickly as I could, Julian Bailes completed several TBI studies at West Virginia University using animals and omega-3s. As I investigated, the truth became clear. Basically we were the only two scientists looking at the nutritional use of omega-3s in the treatment of brain trauma.

According to the Centers for Disease Control and Prevention (CDC), traumatic brain injury is a major cause of death and disability in the United States, contributing to about 30 percent of all injury deaths. Every day, 138 people in the US die from injuries that include traumatic brain injury. In 2010, about 2.5 million emergency department visits, hospitalizations, or deaths were associated with traumatic brain injury, and of that, a large number of those victims were children. This is a big problem.

People in the Army will tell you, "You'll know when it's time to retire when it's time." To this point in my thirty-one-year career, I had always had interesting and enjoyable assignments. But I knew it was time and that I had bigger and more important things I wanted to do. I had put enough time in so that I could retire as a Colonel, and so on January 1, 2012, I hung up my uniform and began a nonprofit called the Brain Health Education and Research Institute (BHERI). From the very beginning, the Institute's purpose has been to pursue educational and research endeavors to further our knowledge of natural and nutritional ways to improve brain health. The initial focus of the Institute is educating providers and the public on the use of omega-3 fatty acids for the prevention, treatment, and rehabilitation of the brain prior to or following injury, such as traumatic brain injury or concussion.

BHERI began by trying to develop a professional network focused on learning about omega-3s and developing tools and protocols to help patients find the resources for a nutritional approach to brain trauma. BHERI is a continuation of the work and research I was performing in the military. Ultimately, the Institute's purpose is to educate people on why omega-3s are so crucial to brain health and brain injuries, and hopefully to foster or even fund research in the area and move the science further along. That takes money and, unfortunately, donations have been few and far between.

The grapevine in science and medicine is fast and strong, and suddenly friends, friends of friends, and then strangers began contacting me looking for help with treating concussion. One good friend urged me to set up a website to make The Omega Protocols available to everyone, and another friend helped set up the site. Before we knew it, the BHERI website was seeing over one thousand hits a day from people seeking information for their loved ones suffering from a brain injury. Athletic directors from university sports programs initiated contact. Anguished parents sent emails and phoned in about their sons and daughters. Coaches asked about concussion prevention. But the basic, most important question parents, coaches, and some doctors were asking was simple: "What can I do?"

Today there are more than two million concussions a year in children. Most concussion injuries do not show up on CT scans. In more severe concussion, debilitating effects of brain trauma often go untreated. I spent the last decade seeking answers to the question Bobby's anguished father asked me over the phone, "Isn't there something, anything, more we can do?"

Yes. There is more you can do.

CHAPTER ONE

CHILD'S PLAY, YOUTH IN SPORTS

Julian Bailes was played by Alec Baldwin in *Concussion*, the Columbia Pictures film starring Will Smith as forensic pathologist Dr. Bennet Omalu, who ends up exposing the real, persistent dangers of concussion and his attempts to bring the issue to the NFL. In the film, as in real life, Bailes is Omalu's ally. *Concussion*, numerous documentaries, ongoing research, articles, and books have all exposed the health risks of head strikes and brain trauma associated with playing football. But the issues surrounding concussion, especially in youth sports, are also pervasive, widespread, and not limited to football—concussion is a crisis.

Out of the 3 to 4.5 million concussions every year, nearly 2,000,000 are children aged nineteen or younger who are treated in emergency rooms for sports and recreational related injuries for concussion. The list for sports-related brain trauma includes soccer, hockey, lacrosse, wrestling, playgrounds, bicycles, skateboards, horseback riding, and falls. Though this number of reported sports-related concussions is sobering, it is almost ancillary compared to the millions of concussions in children that go unreported. One spring, the parents of one of those children came to me.

On May 5, 2013, I received an email from the father of a thirteen-year-old baseball player. Justin had been struck in the head, beamed, by a fastball, and then picked himself up, dusted himself off, and took first base. His father had been a triple-A baseball player who was injured himself just as he was called up to the Florida Marlins, and his career never launched. Now, years later, he was a father. His son, Justin, and my son played several sports, including baseball, together when they were kids. At one point, I was the baseball coach and Justin was on my team, which is kind of a joke because Dad obviously knew a lot more about baseball than I did. I never made it past Little League.

I knew the boy, I knew the family, and they were our friends. Justin had come home from the game that Saturday, after getting hit by that pitch, with a very minor headache and took a nap. Other than being sleepy, he didn't show any symptoms. On Sunday, he played again in the afternoon, and his dad recognized that he made several uncharacteristically bad decisions. The head-ache returned in the evening after the game, and he was exhausted. He still didn't seem to have any other symp-toms other than fatigue and headache. The father reached out to me because he knew I was involved in brain injury studies and I was a past coach. They never took Justin to the ER, but assumed he had suffered a mild concussion. I explained how rest was really important, that electronics and any activity that might further stress Justin's brain needed to be limited, but I also told the father to buy fish oil and start The Omega-3 Protocol immediately. Justin was to take five capsules that night, five with breakfast, and then five capsules three times a day for the next week.

They began the protocol that evening. On the first full day, the intensity of Justin's headache lessened by the afternoon. On Tuesday, the second day after the injury, he was able to go to school all day. Though the headache was pretty much gone, he took a nap as soon as he came home. On Wednesday, he only attended a half day of school because he had a school event that night. He rested for two weeks all together, continued with the fish oil, kept to the protocol, and resumed playing baseball fourteen days after the concussion. Justin now takes fish oil every day, and his energy level and brain function is normal. It is my hope that he will continue to take fish oil to strengthen his brain's inner armor. Fish oil and omega-3s can also serve in a preventive role.

Forty-four million children play organized sports in the United States. We know there are 1.1 million high school football players alone with another 1.1 million kids playing pre-high school, youth football. In addition, more than 3 million to 4 million kids are registered with US youth soccer leagues. Of the two of these sports, the largest number of youth concussions are from boys' high school football. The second largest number are from girls' high school soccer. Of those two populations, girls tend to suffer the worst. Youth girls' concussions are more complicated and they don't recover as quickly. There is speculation as to why, but answers are slow in coming.

The question arises as to whether concussion is on the rise. There is definitely an increase in concussions reported. The question is whether it's a true increase or if it's just that the awareness has created the increase, a phenomena known as "surveillance bias." Parents and coaches are more aware, so they're more apt to report an injury, pull a child from a game, and notify health-care professionals. I think there probably are more concussions, but there's also certainly much more awareness, and that's one of the positive outcomes from the NFL's discussion around brain injury and helmets. That narrative has created a much greater awareness of concussion over the last ten years and translates into an increase in reporting concussions.

Another contributing factor to increases in reporting is simply better technology and better diagnostics. We have better imaging technology and more acute neurological testing, so injuries can be detected. Even then, however, a concussion can go undiagnosed. A CT scan will not pick up most concussions. Neurological testing can lead to a false negative, and though the child may test well, he or she can still be besieged with headaches, irritability, and confusion.

Sports have changed as well. Bigger, stronger, faster players are groomed for longer periods of time, practices take up more days of the week, and players are encouraged to practice hard and play hard. In football, the defensive backs launch themselves at the running backs headfirst in an attempt to hit the running backs as hard as possible and knock them down. The problem is, the running backs are getting bigger and stronger, and now the running backs are bouncing off of the defensive backs. Both can suffer. That form of tackling is becoming less and less effective because of how much bigger and stronger the players have become. The combination of harder play with physically larger kids, coupled with better diagnostics and public awareness, means concussion is more widely reported.

Here's a real-life example. Just two years ago there were zero concussions at my son's high school. Do you believe that? No, I don't believe it either, but that's what the school nurse tells me. She knows that number is not correct either. Last year she dealt with over forty kids with concussions. This year, she's already dealt with twice as many, and we are only halfway through the year. This huge increase is due to better reporting and a new awareness of concussion.

Research continues to develop as well. A recent twelve-point clinical score for children with concussion has been developed and shown to identify those who are more likely to have prolonged symptoms and, therefore, need closer follow-up. The study, published in the *Journal of the American Medical Association* (JAMA), was conducted by a team led by Dr. Roger Zemek, of Children's Hospital of Eastern Ontario Research Institute, Ottawa, Canada. "We have developed an easy-to-calculate clinical score which could potentially individualize concussion care in children, identifying those with high risk of prolonged symptoms who will need closer follow-up," Zemek told *Medscape Medical News*.

"The first question parents ask is, 'When is my child going to be better?' But prior to this work we didn't have any scientific basis to answer this question," he said. Zemek explained how concussion symptoms are often prolonged for more than a month in about one third of cases. One month. Symptoms can include headache, dizziness, and difficulty concentrating, symptoms that have an adverse effect on quality of life and can affect school attendance and exam performance. "Currently we cannot tell which patients are more likely to have prolonged symptoms," Zemek said. "It is important to be able to provide the family with some realistic guidance on when the child is likely to recover and to be able to target specialist care to the higher-risk patients."

Zemek's team of researchers looked at more than seventy possible variables and found nine that seemed to be particularly independently associated with long-term symptoms: female sex, age thirteen years or older, a history of migraine, previous concussion with symptoms lasting longer than a week, headache, sensitivity to noise, fatigue, answering questions slowly, and difficulty standing on a balance beam. The researchers developed a scoring system, and their results "suggest that a score of 9 to 12 on this scale signifies a high risk of prolonged symptoms of concussion, with a 93% certainty," Zemek said. "We can also say that a score of 9 to 12 means that a child is three times more likely to have persistent symptoms than the standard score. And a score of 0 to 3 means they are three times less likely than a standard score to have prolonged issues."

Justin, the thirteen-year-old baseball player, was one of those kids whose concussion was never reported. No one was scoring his fatigue level or testing balance, but his parents rightly assumed he suffered a minor concussion. So what can a parent or a coach do to help a child who has suffered a concussion? Why does The Omega-3

Protocol work? How does it help? Are there preventive measures that can be taken? Why is the brain so susceptible to concussion?

BRAIN FOOD: YOU ARE WHAT YOU EAT

The answers are in the science of the brain. The brain is made of fat, and about 30 percent of that fat is what are called omega-3 fatty acids. Omega-3s have many important, critical functions. The concept of The Omega-3 Protocol is that if we saturate the brain with what it is made of, and we help create the nutritional foundation for the brain to heal, it will heal.

Think of a brick wall. If you have a brick wall that gets damaged, you probably want to use bricks to repair the wall. Omega-3s are, literally, the bricks of the brain. Omega-3s make up a significant part of every neuron cell membrane. There is no cure for concussion and TBI. There are no magic medicines, nor will there ever be. The brain must heal itself. But what we can do is optimize the conditions to help the brain do the healing. That is what using omega-3s will do. They provide a tool, the basic building block, for the brain to recover.

It would be great if we all ate enough foods high in omega-3s, but we don't. The problem is that omega-6 fatty acids are even more abundant in nature and in our food supply. While omega-3s are anti-inflammatory and pro-resolving, increase blood flow, and enhance the immune system, omega-6s promote inflammation, increase blood clotting, and depress the immune system.

Humans evolved consuming a diet that contained approximately equal amounts of omega-3 and omega-6 fatty acids. About a hundred years ago, the industrial revolution introduced technology that refined vegetable oils. At the same time, there was a meteoric rise in the production and consumption of processed foods. Both led to a dramatic increase in the consumption of omega-6 fatty acids.

In addition, the introduction of animal feeds derived from grains rich in omega-6 fats has resulted in the production of meat, fish, and eggs high in omega-6 fatty acids and virtually devoid of omega-3 fatty acids. Today, in Western diets, the ratio of omega-6 to omega-3 fatty acids ranges from 20:1 to 30:1 instead of the pre-industrial range of 1:1 to 2:1. Research has shown that this imbalanced intake of omegas is a contributing factor to many chronic health conditions such as heart disease, diabetes, arthritis, depression, asthma, allergies, and obesity. This imbalance also makes the brain more susceptible to concussion and TBI, and it limits the biochemical ability of the brain to heal itself. As a friend of mine at the NIH says, "Junk food equals junk brain."

Our bodies were meant to be in balance. It gets back to what you should have learned in kindergarten, and the concept is simple: You are what you eat.

Both the American diet and the American food supply have changed dramatically in the last fifty years. During World War II, we saved the world from tyranny. In subsequent decades, we eliminated polio, developed vaccines and antibiotics, and even landed a man on the moon! There was nothing that couldn't be conquered, so how could we have starving children in America? The answer was found in farm subsidies and food programs that started in the 1960s and 1970s. Soybean and corn are calorie-dense, shelf-stable, easy-to-grow crops that were subsidized by the government. As a result, the amount of soybean consumption by the United States population has grown exponentially.

The biggest source of omega-6s in the American diet today is soybean oil. Its consumption has gone up 1600 percent since 1970. Soybean oil is shelf-stable, so processed food is often rich in omega-6s. In contrast, omega-3s spoil very easily, so food additives rich in omega-3s are not used by the food industry. The food industry isn't intentionally trying to harm people; rather, the industry is focused on making food more shelf-stable so it can be shipped cross-country and sit on grocery store shelves for long periods of time. The result, however, is that soy and omega-6s are in everything, particularly processed foods.

The result has been a growing imbalance between omega-6s and omega-3s in the food chain and subsequently in our brains. Omega-6s are critical for brain development

OILSEEDS IN THE US FOOD SUPPLY

MODIFIED FROM Blasbalg et al., Am. J. Clin. Nutr. 93: 950–962, 2011

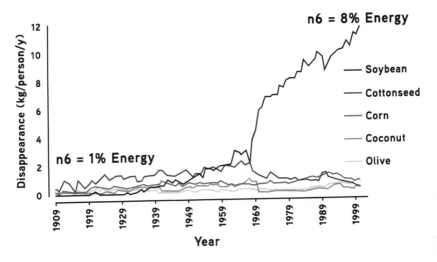

and function, but they are also very pro-inflammatory. Inflammation is a crucial process to fight infections and bring healing to an infected or injured part of the body. Omega-3s are equally critical and serve as balance with anti-inflammatory and pro-resolving properties. But in the last half century, the foods we eat have set the balance between the pro- and anti-inflammatory omega-6 and omega-3s off-kilter. We have way too many omega-6s in our diet and in our brains.

Now the preconditions are set for additional trauma when the brain is injured. If there is a head injury, the brain is flooded with inflammatory factors from omega-6s, which is necessary, to a point. We need inflammatory responses to address the injury, but we also need the anti-inflammatory and pro-resolving omega-3s to calm the brain and extinguish the fire of inflammation. If that doesn't occur, the acute injury can turn into a situation of chronic inflammation that continues to burn for weeks, months, or even years.

One of the pressing questions is: Does this imbalance make us more susceptible to getting a concussion? We don't know for sure, but certainly if a concussion occurs, a person may have more symptoms or the damage may be worse because of the imbalance between the omega-6s and omega-3s.

What the brain needs, especially during trauma, is a balance between the omega-6s and omega-3s. Fish oil, filled with omega-3s, provides this protective armor and helps feed the brain with what it needs to heal. To be clear, omega-3s are not some miracle drug. They are nutrition. When administered as a nutritional supplement in a protocol for TBI and concussion, they will only help heal the brain as much as it can be healed. Sometimes the damage is too great and nothing will help. Often, however, this healing far exceeds the expectations of doctors, parents, coaches, and patients. What we need to focus on is building that inner armor of omega-3s in our young players.

SHOULD MY CHILD STOP PLAYING TEAM SPORTS?

Because I study TBI and concussions, have been a sports coach, and sit on advisory panels for youth sports, I am routinely asked, "Should kids stop playing sports?" And my answer is always no. An emphatic *no*.

I'm a huge fan of team sports. I played all kinds of sports growing up. As kids, when we weren't playing on a team, we were playing pickup games around the neighborhood. We were constantly outside and playing any sport that involved a ball. I played football from the age of nine or ten up through freshman year of college, and then I switched over to rugby and played rugby through college and beyond. My children play team sports. The importance of exercise should not be minimized by fear.

The values children draw from team sports are twofold. There's the intrinsic value of leadership and cooperation. Life is a team sport, and what better way to learn life lessons than on the field playing team sports? You learn how to be a member of a team, how to persevere, how to win and lose graciously, how to be a leader and how to follow, and how to work together as a team. Football, in particular, is interesting in that, yes, it is rough and violent, but every player on the field has an important role on every play. It's not just the player with the ball that is important. Every player is important. If even one player on the team lets down and misses a block or a tackle, the whole team is affected, maybe even the outcome of the game. All those are lessons you need for a good life, and we should be learning them on the sports fields as youths. You're not going to learn them as an adult in the workforce. If that's where you're trying to learn them, you're probably already too late, or, at the very least, you have a lot of social catching up to do.

When I was a cadet at West Point, as part of the first-year initiation we had to memorize a lot of things about the history of West Point and the Army. One of those things was a quotation by General Douglas MacArthur when he was Superintendent at West Point a century ago. He knew the value of team sports. He said:

"Upon the fields of friendly strife are sown the seeds that upon other fields on other days, will bear the fruits of victory."

In addition to the intrinsic values of playing team sports is the physical value of exercise. Obesity in the US is a bigger problem than concussions. We need kids to be outside playing sports, being active, cooperating, and feeling proud of the team and their bodies. This is true for adults as well. What's the alternative? You certainly don't learn the values of leadership and cooperation or tone your body from sitting on the couch playing video games.

Then comes the next tier of concerns and attempts at regulating youth sports: perhaps youth football should just be banned—or girls soccer. But if you ban football or soccer, then it is a matter of time before the spotlight shines on the next sport. It's an absurd argument that we should ban any popular sport that gets kids off the couch and on the field. What we need to do is realize that the benefits of team sports like football and soccer far outweigh the risks of those sports—but we need to get better at mitigating the risks, by making the sports safer.

MAKING THE FIELD SAFER

There are three ways to make team sports safer. One is to craft rules of game play that enhance safer play and then enforce those rules. The second is to reduce contact during practice. The third is to develop rules around specific techniques that are allowed based on the maturity of the player.

To illustrate the importance of enforcing rules of the game, let's look at "Targeting" in football. Targeting is the practice of leading with your head, and it's supposed to be a penalty at all levels of play, whether enforced or not. The NCAA, the college football league, will review a play if it's questionable and throw the player out during the game if the penalty is considered flagrant. The same rule applies in college basketball. In the National Football League, this practice is not replicated. The game continues, spectators watch, and it seems as though nothing punitive happens beyond a fifteen-yard penalty. The league just fines the player $10,000 and a kid watching in the stands or on television has no concept of any punitive action. The fine is a drop in the bucket for these guys. The NFL ought to throw the offending player out of the game immediately and show younger players that targeting will not be tolerated on the field. This policy of player removal ought to be enforced at all levels of football, whether it's youth football or the NFL. Adults, as always, should be setting the example.

The second way to reduce concussion in collision sports is to eliminate contact during practices as much as practical. The idea is if we just decrease the potential for contact, logically there are less opportunities for collisions, which then translates into less cases of concussion. By removing opportunity, we decrease the risk of long-term problems. The film *Concussion* makes reference to the fact that over the career of Pittsburgh Steeler Hall of Fame Center Mike Webster, taking into account all his years of playing from childhood through to retirement from the NFL, suffered as many as 70,000 strikes to the head if not more. This means Webster suffered 70,000 subconcussive strikes to his skull and brain, yet he was never once diagnosed with having a concussion. Now this is an educated estimate to be sure; there's no way to actually measure that number. But if you could decrease that total, even by a third, then the potential exists to decrease the chances of incurring long-term neurological injury. Not every strike to the head leads to a concussion, but each time the brain gets rattled, it sets off an inflammatory cascade. If the brain loses its ability to clear up that inflammation, the long-term damage may be seen in increased rates of chronic traumatic encephalopathy, or CTE, or other neurologic diseases that are higher in football players, boxers, and other collision-sport athletes.

The official name for Pop Warner Football is Pop Warner Little Scholars, and there are roughly 325,000 kids in the organization from ages five to sixteen. In 2010, Pop Warner established a medical advisory committee led by Julian Bailes, and I was asked to serve. One of the first measures we offered as decreasing the potential for concussion injuries was a reduction in the number of practices involving contact. This meant the number of hours and number of practices could remain the same, but actual contact would be reduced. How to do it was the question. Enforcing it is yet another question. The answer really is that there needs to be a strong effort to educate the coaches.

Coaches at the college level certainly are aware of the concussion crisis. The University of Alabama instituted a no-hitting policy after the beginning of the season. We asked Nick Saban, the head coach of the University of Alabama football team, to speak to the Pop Warner Youth Football Medical Advisory Committee. Saban explained how he led his team, Crimson Tide, to win four national championships in seven years. Yet, Coach Saban enforces a policy of absolutely zero contact in practice after the beginning of the season.

Saban explained to the Pop Warner Committee that

he does not allow any contact during practice after the beginning of the season because he doesn't want to risk a player suffering a concussion or other injury and missing a game because he can't play. As a result of research, Saban's talk, and growing concern over concussion, Pop Warner Football made changes to their practice regime for K–12 children. Coaches now operate under the following guidelines:

1. No full-speed head-on blocking or tackling drills in which the players line up more than three yards apart are permitted. Having two linemen in stances immediately across the line of scrimmage from each other and having full-speed drills where the players approach each other at an angle, but not straight ahead in to each other, are both permitted. However, there should be no intentional head-to-head contact.

2. The amount of contact at each practice will be reduced to a maximum of one-third of practice time (either forty minutes total of each practice or one-third of total weekly practice time). In this context, *contact* means any drill or scrimmage, including down-line vs. down-line full-speed drills.

In 2012, Pop Warner, the largest youth football organization in the country, established this limited contact rule. Here, adults modeled correct team behavior for kids.

Recently, in March 2016, all eight Ivy League football

teams voted unanimously to eliminate contact in football practices after the beginning of the season. This follows in the footsteps of one of their own, Dartmouth College. Dartmouth football coach Buddy Teevens decided in 2010 to eliminate all full-contact practices throughout the entire year, including pre-season, in an effort to reduce injuries. Teevens makes a promise to recruited players before they take the field: "In four years, you will never tackle another Dartmouth football player." Dartmouth has seen a big decrease in concussions that kept players out of games and injuries that wore the team down over the course of a season.

The University of New Hampshire went a step further and now practices tackling without helmets so players learn to keep their heads out of the way. They then tracked players' injuries in a scientific study. Players who participated in the no-helmet training experienced 28 percent fewer head impacts in games at the end of the season compared to the control group. Sean McDonnell, the head coach at New Hampshire, says no-contact practice taught his players "not to use the helmet as a weapon. What's happened is that the helmet is so well designed that kids feel they couldn't get hurt no matter what."

These decisions by teams and leagues to limit contact during practice could and should influence how other football programs, from youth to professional, try to mitigate the physical toll of football and lower the risk of concussion. Remember, the most debilitating consequences of concussions in sports are often not the result of one single blow, but a series of subconcussive strikes to the head over time.

The third way to reduce concussion is to limit what the head can take, in terms of the age of the athlete and the strength of the neck, and modify training. For example, US Soccer has banned all heading, whether in practice or in games, for youth under the age of eleven. In hockey there's body checking, when a player has the puck and, if you're a defender, you can physically ram into the player and knock the other player down or knock him into the boards. It's essentially a tackle on ice. The USA Hockey organization has now stated that body checking is prohibited for players twelve and under. The even better news is that they're actually talking about proposing to move the age up to fourteen.

These are examples of strategies in several sports that will reduce the possibility of head injury—if these rules and strategies are enforced. Couple these with good public education around these measures, and there would be fewer head injuries and fewer concussions. The strategy to reducing the number and severity of concussions should be the use of reasonable caution, not banning team sports for youth.

A child should play smart and be coached smart. This includes playing hard when the body is developed enough to handle certain moves and plays in practice and on the field. Archie Manning was a professional football player, a quarterback, mostly known for playing on the New Orleans Saints in the 1960s and early 1970s. At the time, he was considered one of the better quarterbacks in the league, but the New Orleans Saints were not a strong team, so his potential was never realized. After his almost-spectacular career, Manning went on to father three sons. Though they all played football, the oldest one had a medical issue with his neck that forced him to stop playing in college, as he ran the risk of being paralyzed. The second brother, Peyton Manning, and the youngest son, Eli Manning, are currently quarterbacks in the NFL. More impressive is the fact that both of them have won the Super Bowl. Twice.

Peyton Manning is, arguably, the most talented quarterback in the history of football. He has been voted MVP of the league five times. He just won the Super Bowl in 2016 for the second time and he's announced that he has retired. It's interesting that you have two quarterbacks who are brothers who have won the Super Bowl four times between the two of them. Both will probably be honored in the league's Hall of Fame. And here's the kicker: they did not play tackle football until seventh grade!

Another one of the greatest quarterbacks is Tom Brady of the New England Patriots. His father didn't allow him to play tackle football until ninth grade.

Peyton Manning and Tom Brady are phenomenal players, yet they didn't play tackle football until they were teens. Tom Brady's father has said in hindsight, "I'd be very hesitant to let my son play at all today, given what I've learned about concussions."

This willingness to hold back, to not allow certain types of game play or practice routines until a child is older and neck muscles are developed enough, is key to preventing concussion. You don't have to play tackle football in kindergarten to be an MVP.

CHAPTER TWO

ADULT INJURIES

WHO GETS HURT

Kelly was a forty-three-year-old woman who worked from home. One morning after dropping her daughter off at school, she was sitting at a traffic light waiting for the light to turn green when, suddenly, she was thrown violently forward. Another woman, who was texting while driving, struck Kelly's car at fifty miles per hour. Though shaken, Kelly felt fine and shrugged off transport to the hospital. Her car was totaled, but again, she felt fine. She had a friend pick her up at the scene of the accident. But on the drive home, Kelly began to feel ill and told her friend to take her to the emergency room.

Over the next month, Kelly went to the ER three times for symptoms of concussion from the accident. What most people do not realize is that concussion unfolds in two phases. The first phase is the primary injury, where the brain tissues are violently thrown against the inside of the skull, whether because the head hit the windshield or because of helmet-to-helmet contact on the football field, a soccer ball strike, or a fall. The primary injury changes the way the brain functions, and brings about a secondary injury which can be far more devastating: a biochemical cascade triggered by the initial impact that can go on for months and create dangerous conditions in the brain, such as oxygen deprivation and inflammation, or excess fluid in the cranium. That's why victims of concussion can die a week or two after an initial head injury. It's also why symptoms can linger even in a mild concussion.

When I was introduced to Kelly, five weeks had elapsed since she pulled up to that light. I did a thorough evaluation including a detailed mapping of her brain and began seeing her as a patient. She was suffering from memory loss and brain fog. "Brain fog" is just what it sounds like. Though not a medical term, it describes feelings of confusion and the lack of focus and mental clarity patients can suffer from when brain function is impaired. Kelly said she didn't remember anything about what she did for the month or so after the accident. But she was used to memory lapses and brain fog. Three years before she was rear-ended, she was involved in another car accident—a head-on collision. This accident resulted in a concussion as well. I saw her after her second car accident, her second concussion in three years.

Now she was left moody and emotionally volatile. She had difficulty sleeping. She couldn't participate in simple activities with her daughter. If they settled in for the evening and tried to watch a movie, Kelly couldn't tolerate the interaction of watching TV with her daughter. She also couldn't remember much of the month that followed her accident.

The first thing I did was start Kelly on high doses of fish oil.

A month into the nutritional therapy, her symptoms dissipated. Kelly could sleep through the night, she was able to stay focused, and the brain fog had lifted. She felt more like herself again. On one follow-up visit, her thirteen-year-old daughter came along. After she and her mother settled into chairs, her daughter turned to me and said, "Thank you. You gave me my mom back." I only wish I could do this for every patient and their families.

WHO GETS HURT ON THE FIELD

Brain concussion can happen anywhere, at any time. In Kelly's case, she had no idea she was going to get rear-ended. Statistically, the leading cause of traumatic brain injury is falls. More than half of traumatic brain injuries in children are caused by falls. Eighty percent of head injuries in adults, age sixty-five and older, are caused by falls. Often the spotlight is on the NFL and the military, but the problem of head injury is much larger. Even when the number of NFL players with TBI and the number of military personnel with TBI are combined, this number pales in comparison to the number of TBI sufferers in the general population. In 2010, there were about 2.5 million emergency department visits, hospitalizations, or deaths associated with head injuries.

I was often criticized by some of my military physician colleagues for my focus on concussion. They couldn't understand why I focused on sports concussions when head injuries in the military are such a visible challenge. The facts are clear, however. In ten years of being at war in the Middle East, there have only been 20,000 recorded TBIs. Though tragic, this number is dwarfed by the 2.5 million reported concussions *a year* not associated with the military that are injuries resulting from sports and other accidents.

The flood of media attention highlighting damaged brains, dementia, and suicides in retired NFL players has made concussions synonymous with football. That attention was greatly needed, as the debilitating consequences of brain injuries in football players of all ages have been severely overlooked. But the focus of this controversy has been far too narrow. Believe it or not, equestrian sports have the highest rate of head injuries of all sports.

In addition, in many of the most popular sports, boys aren't the ones most likely to be afflicted by concussions—

girls are. Across all sports in a study, the highest rate of concussion was reported not by male football players, but by female ice hockey players. There are not as many players as men's football, but the percentage of players to rates of concussion is larger. This is important to note because recent studies of high school and college athletes have shown that girls and women suffer from concussions at higher rates than their male counterparts in similar sports. This gender disparity holds true for baseball/softball, soccer, basketball, and lacrosse.

For instance, in a recent analysis of college athletic injuries, female softball players experienced concussions at double the rate of male baseball players. Women also experienced higher rates of concussions than men in basketball and soccer. Female ice hockey players experienced a concussion once every 1,100 games or practices—nearly three times the rate experienced in football.

The gender disparity exists in high school sports, too. One study, analyzing concussion data for athletes in twenty-five high schools, found that in soccer girls experienced concussions at twice the rate of boys. We have some evidence that the brains of female athletes are more susceptible—or, at least, react differently—to injury compared to their male counterparts. It may be the interplay with hormone levels, or it might be that girls' neck muscles are not as well developed and make their heads more susceptible to concussions. We need to stop assuming concussion is a men's issue. We shouldn't simply accept that the best practices for boys' and men's sports will protect girls and women in the same way. The bodies of female athletes are different, and their brains deserve just as much attention.

I bring this up not to encourage parents of girls to forbid their daughters to play team sports, but to point out that coaches and parents may not think of concussion as a statistical reality for their young players. What happens in the adult world is mirrored in youth sports and is just as important to recognize, try to prevent, and treat.

THE IMPORTANCE OF PREVENTION AND OMEGA-3S

If your child or a loved one is diagnosed with concussion or you suspect concussion, every medical textbook, website, and health-care provider is going to tell you the same thing:

- Get plenty of rest.
- Avoid physical activities and sports while in recovery.
- See your health-care provider, who may prescribe medicine if symptoms such as a headache, difficulty sleeping, or depression persist.

[www.cdc.gov/headsup/basics/concussion_recovery.html]

These measures are important. However, no current therapies address either the secondary phase that continues to damage the brain over the hours and days following injury, or the need to facilitate the early neuroregeneration process to help the brain repair damage. In reality, many children and patients with brain trauma and concussion are not assessed nutritionally at all. Yet, when tracked, children with severe head injuries who are given early nutritional support are associated with better outcomes and less mortality.

"What is exciting about our findings is that kids seemed to have a better outcome, both with respect to mortality and to functional outcomes, if they were fed within seventy-two hours of being in the ICU," said Elizabeth Meinert, MD, from the University of Pittsburgh Medical Center. "There are a lot of high-tech and physiology-focused treatments for TBI, and I think that sometimes we forget about feeding these kids because we're so worried about their brains," she told Medscape Medical News. "It's important to remember that nutrition is another treatment for the brain," Dr. Meinert went on to say at the Society of Critical Care Medicine's 45th Critical Care Congress.

In their study of TBI patients requiring hospitalization, the timing of nutritional support varied widely. It was found that 35.5% of the children received nutritional support forty-eight hours or less after the TBI, 40.0% received it forty-eight to seventy-two hours after the injury, 18.9% received it more than seventy-two hours after the injury, and 5.6% received no nutritional support during the study period. The mortality rate was significantly higher in children who did not receive any nutritional support than in those who did, and outcomes were significantly worse.

"There's an increasing focus on good nutrition in ICUs and, while that's common sense, it's nice to actually have some data to support that we do need to address nutrition early," said Lori Shutter, MD, from the University of Pittsburgh Medical Center, who moderated the oral session. "In managing patients in the ICU, we also need to create an optimum environment to allow some natural healing, and nutrition is a component of that optimal environment that we often overlook." While these doctors were discussing more severe TBI patients who land in ICUs in hospitals around the country, the same holds true for all TBI and concussion patients.

When I retired from the military, and started the Brain Health Education and Research Institute, one of the first events the organization sponsored in June 2012 was a conference called *Advances in the Prevention and Management of Sports Related Concussions*. The conference hosted speakers from the CDC, the NIH, the University of Pittsburgh, the Pittsburgh Steeler football team, and Julian Bailes, Professor, Chair of Neurosurgery, North-Shore University HealthSystem, University of Chicago (by then, Dr. Bailes had left West Virginia University). The conference was formed to look at preventive interventions that could be practically applied to both the military and team sports and gave recommendations for coaches and medical professionals to follow once concussion is suspected or diagnosed.

One of the outcomes was the suggestion that athletes and soldiers should take omega-3s preventively, in preparation of potential injury. Because of our collaborative work, Dr. Bailes and I had just published a paper in *Military Medicine* in 2011 looking at exactly that issue: using fish oil as a way to protect the brain from potential injury. The journal article, "Neuro-protection for the Warrior: Dietary Supplementation with Omega-3 Fatty Acids," advocated that people who are at risk or high exposure to brain injury, such as soldiers and athletes, ought to be taking fish oil supplementation on a daily basis.

Our paper pointed out that nutrition has traditionally involved supplying energy and hydration. What is emerging from research is the concept of using omega-3 fatty acids to increase the resilience of the brain prior to injury. Omega-3s have numerous proven benefits in support of cardiovascular and psychiatric health. Omega-3s provide benefits by exerting a protective mechanism at the cellular and neuronal levels including calming the inflammatory cascade following traumatic brain injury.

Then we made a more profound claim: "More exciting is that new laboratory research demonstrates beneficial effects extend to when omega-3s are given before injury. Given the safety profile, availability, and affordability of fish oil, Generally Recognized As Safe amounts of ... fish oil (3,000 milligrams/day of combined EPA and DHA) should be considered for the athlete and soldier, not only for general health benefits, but particularly also for those at risk or high exposure to brain impacts. A comprehensive, coordinated research program to evaluate the multiple uses of omega-3 fatty acids should be a high priority for the Department of Defense.

"Promising research and evolving clinical experience now indicate omega-3s are useful and effective for recovery following TBI and concussion. New laboratory research shows the beneficial effects extend to when omega-3s are given prior to injury. Given the safety profile, availability, and affordability of omega-3s, it should be considered a beneficial supplement for the athlete and soldier, not only for its general health benefits, but particularly for those at risk of high exposure to brain impacts. Based upon current knowledge and experience, omega-3s should be consumed at already FDA-approved doses of 3 grams per day in soft gels (typically 5 capsules of quality concentrated fish oil) to increase the resiliency of the brain to withstand injury."

In other words, fish oil may help prevent concussion in the first place!

The FDA carries a standard of measurement called GRAS, which stands for Generally Recognized as Safe. Currently, the FDA recognizes 3,000 milligrams of combined EPA and DHA omega-3s as Generally Recognized as

Safe (GRAS). Dr. Bailes and I took the position and made the recommendation that soldiers and athletes who are at risk of head injuries and concussions should be taking the FDA Generally Recognized as Safe dose of 3,000 milligrams of combined EPA and DHA a day—every day.

The question, then, poses itself. If omega-3s help with healing the brain and can be used to prevent or lessen the effects of concussion, do omega-3s have any impact on brain trauma that occurred months or, in some cases, even years ago? To find the answer, the first place I looked was a pool of patients who had suffered many subconcussive strikes to the head over time. They were also easily accessible patients to study: retired NFL players.

In 1976, Randy Cross was selected in the second round of the NFL draft by the San Francisco 49ers. His thirteen-year career included six all-pro selections, three pro-bowl selections, and three Super Bowl championships during the Joe Montana era. Since his retirement from the NFL, Randy has re-created himself as a radio and TV personality and commentator, and he has appeared or carried shows on NBC and CBS Sports.

I was introduced to him a few years ago through a mutual friend. Randy told me he felt like he was having some cognitive issues. I started him on high-dose omega-3s. This was 2012, and his last game in the NFL had been Super Bowl XXIII in 1989. He was suffering from what I've seen in several NFL players: a lack of energy, overwhelming fatigue, brain fog, and not thinking clearly. So I started him on The Omega Protocol, on the high doses of fish oil, fifteen capsules of fish oil per day.

Randy noticed an improvement in his energy levels and cognitive ability and a decrease in brain fog within a couple of days. It took less than a week for Randy to feel the effects of the omega-3s. In an email he wrote, "I have noticed a bit of difference in mental quickness after the third day."

In May 2012, a very popular football player named Junior Seau committed suicide. Suicide among veterans and retired sports players is higher with those who suffered past concussion and depression is a very real and insidious complication of concussion. It has been estimated that twenty-two veterans commit suicide every day, and there have been a number of high-profile former NFL players who have committed suicide. Seau was only forty-three years-old.

As a precaution, I checked in with Randy to see how he was doing and if he was continuing to use omega-3s. We spoke on the phone, and he was amazed by how clear-headed he was and the increase in his energy level.

Randy went on enthusiastically and explained how he was still taking ten to fifteen capsules a day because, he said, "I like how it makes me feel." If he was traveling for work and forgot to throw a bottle of fish oil in his bag, he discovered his energy level decreased and the brain fog returned over a few days. When that happened, he didn't think twice. He'd scout around and find a health-food store and stock up with another bottle of fish oil. By morning he'd be himself again. He joked that he was accumulating bottles of fish oil from around the country.

The question of using omega-3s as treatment for older brain injuries and for immediate concussion and as a preventive prophylactic will be explored later in the book. The Omega Protocol is not a medical intervention or treatment. It is a nutritional approach, based in scientific research that supports brain function and helps the brain recover from trauma by supplying the brain the food it needs to protect itself and heal.

CHAPTER THREE

REINFORCING THE INNER ARMOR

THE IMPORTANCE OF OMEGA-3 FATTY ACIDS

CONCUSSION CHOWDER

Missy Chase Lapine is also known as the Sneaky Chef. She has made it her business to teach parents how to put healthy foods into meals without their children sniffing out the affronting ingredients. She's learned how to blend vegetables into a red sauce for spaghetti, how to make "brainy brownies," and how to create real nutrition-value breakfast bars.

Over the last couple of years, we had become good friends after being introduced one New Year's Eve at a mutual friend's dinner party. She was in the process of publishing yet another book when she contacted me. Her daughter, Samantha, had fallen and hit her head playing touch football and had been diagnosed with a mild concussion. Her symptoms did not clear up, however, and Missy sought my expertise. Here's what unfolded, as Missy reported on *Huffington Post*:

"My 11-year-old daughter, Samantha ("Sammy," as we call her), had fallen and hit her head on the pavement while playing touch football at recess. I asked all the questions moms ask—is she OK, how serious do you think the injury is? ...Sammy [grew] increasingly dizzy, nauseated, confused ... and complained of wicked headaches. She couldn't concentrate. And her vision became so blurred that she couldn't read a word. Her doctor diagnosed her with a mild concussion and prescribed both physical rest and 'cognitive rest' for two weeks...

"What made the biggest difference, however: Her diet. A few days into Sammy's recovery, I remembered my New Year's Eve dinner partner, Dr. Michael Lewis, a physician who, after retiring recently following a career in the Army, started the Brain Health Education and Research Institute to continue his work on the role of omega-3s and concussions. Michael makes the case that omega-3s are the foundation of the brain and, if they are essential for the brain to develop, maybe they would help the brain heal when it gets damaged. There's some evidence that healthy doses of it may reduce inflammation in the brain and could even help it recover faster from an injury. Omega-3s are good for so many other reasons, anyway—like heart health and mood—that I thought why not give it a shot.

"I mashed sardines into Sammy's beloved tuna salad. They don't really alter the flavor, but they do boost—by a ton—the amount of Omega-3s you get from just the tuna (while reducing the mercury). I fed her edamame, put extra beans and veggies in the muffins we baked, and sprinkled flax seed on her morning cereal—all foods rich in Omega-3s fats. And I whipped up a batch of what I dubbed 'concussion chowder,' made with clams, sardines, broth and veggies.

"Within seven days Sammy felt better, and by day ten she was able to read again. The doctor had told me the symptoms would probably last two weeks— and that Sammy wouldn't be able to read or concentrate until the tail end of that time. I have no way of knowing for sure if Omega-loading my daughter helped her recover as fast as she did. But I believe it did make a big impact. I'd tell any parent to give it a try. At the very least, you'll have a kid who is happier and heart-healthier. And who doesn't want that?"

Missy figured out how to get her daughter to consume massive doses of omega-3s by supplementing foods with fatty acids. And she is right that she will never know for sure if the omega-3s in the fish oil and in her "concussion chowder" made a difference. All she knows is her daughter recovered faster than their doctor anticipated and there were no side effects. But the science of omega-3s can lead us to make the claim that the chances the chowder worked are very high.

Omega-3s are a type of fat. Our foods contain three types of energy. You have carbohydrates. You have protein. You have fats. Omega-3s are an important fat that is found naturally in our diet. Omega-3s are polyunsaturated fatty acids, and we have many, many polyunsaturated fats in our food.

These fatty acids have two ends to their molecules. There's a carboxylic acid, which is considered the beginning of the chain—this end is called alpha. The methyl end, which is considered the tail of the chain, is called omega. The nomenclature mirrors the alpha and the omega ends of the Greek alphabet. Ralph Holman (1918–2012) was the scientist who first described these chains, naming them back in the 1930s. He remembered his Sunday school teachings and believed you had to have the beginning and the end named and identified, thus he named them alpha and omega. These ends are important as they allow for additional chains to link together.

There are three types of omega-3 fatty acids critical to human nutrition. There is the alpha linolenic acid (ALA), commonly found in plants such as dark, leafy, green vegetables or flax seed. There is also eicosapentaenoic acid or EPA, as well as docosahexaenoic acid or DHA. Both EPA and DHA are commonly found in, and derived from, seafood and marine sources, though they are found in meat sources on land as well.

Omega-3 fatty acids are important for normal metabolism. Humans and other mammals are unable to synthesize omega-3 fatty acids by themselves, but they can metabolize the shorter, eighteen-carbon chain of ALA, through diet. This shorter chain can then be use to form the longer chains of EPA and DHA. EPA is twenty carbons in length with five double bonds. DHA is twenty-two carbons in length with six double bonds. However, the ability of the human body to make EPA and DHA from ALA is extremely limited. It is estimated that less than 4 percent of ALA will ever get converted to DHA and incorporated into the brain. Therefore, it's important to consume EPA and DHA directly from the food supply. The most important source of EPA and DHA are cold-water, fatty fish, such as salmon and tuna.

Now consider this: the brain is made up of fat. About 30 percent of the weight of the brain, what we would say is the dry weight of the brain, is made up of omega-3 fatty acids, principally DHA. DHA are the bricks of the brain, the building blocks of cell membranes, and are critical to brain development. The question arises: Can't we just take a supplement of DHA? Why do you need EPA? Interestingly, consuming enough EPA has been found to be important in depression and mental health. EPA also is a very powerful antioxidant and anti-inflammatory, relaxing the circulatory system so blood flows deeper into the brain.

It is estimated that it takes twelve weeks of supplementation for DHA to reach saturation in the brain. That's a long time and doesn't explain why people who take my recommended doses of fish oil experience a profound difference in twenty-four hours. I believe their immediate relief is the result of the combined effect of EPA allowing blood flow deeper into the brain, furthering oxygenation, along with bathing the brain with antioxidants.

TWO WAVES OF RESEARCH

In the last fifty years, there have been two waves of research concerning omega-3s and health, one launched by Danish nutritionists, the other by the National Institute of Health. Hans Olaf Bang and Jørn Dyerberg were nutritionists studying the diets of the Inuit, in Greenland. The Inuit's meals consisted mainly of marine mammals and fish and were very high in whale fat and meat. Complicating matters in terms of favorable health outcomes was the disturbing fact that there were virtually no fruits or vegetables on their dinner tables.

In the United States, that type of diet would be seen as a recipe for heart attack. But the opposite proved true.

There was very little cardiovascular disease among the Inuit. The researchers drew blood from 130 natives and compared their blood reports to Danes. The Inuit had lower levels of lipids such as cholesterol and triglycerides and a higher proportion omega-3 fatty acids. It was discovered that these levels were the result of the consumption of omega-3s in their marine diet. This study began a trail of evidence demonstrating that omega-3s may lower triglycerides, reduce inflammation, and prevent irregular heart rhythms, all of which are believed to be important to heart health.

About twenty years ago, some researchers at the NIH, in particular the National Institute of Alcohol and Alcohol Abuse (NIAAA), started to look at growing evidence that omega-3 fatty acids were related to mental health. Population data was now easier to compile and facts were at their fingertips. Finding correlations between diet and mortality rates and rates of disease became a number-crunching exercise. What they discovered was that populations that had higher consumptions of omega-3s, such as Iceland and Japan, also had much lower rates of mental-health disorders including suicide, depression, and anxiety, as well as lower rates of heart attacks. Further research has shown a positive correlation between omega-3s and reducing the symptoms and negative behaviors of patients with mental-health diseases, ADHD, and autism.

WHAT IS THE DIFFERENCE BETWEEN OMEGA-3 AND OMEGA-6 FATTY ACIDS?

Both omega-3 fatty acids and omega-6 fatty acids are "essential." That's why on food labels you are likely to read "essential fatty acids." Here "essential fatty acids" means these acids are important for health and must be consumed through our diets.

Omega-6s are critical for brain development and function, hormone production, and muscle growth. Some of the downstream effects of arachidonic acid, in particular, include inflammation, which sounds negative but is actually necessary for healing, promoting blood clotting, increasing cell proliferation, and depressing the immune system. Pain and inflammation is a necessary signal for the body to repair itself. Pain is an important indicator preventing further injury, and inflammation is a trigger for our immune system. But too much inflammation or chronic inflammation is hard on the body and can set up a precondition where a trigger can cause a biochemical cascade that keeps repeating an inflammatory cycle. There are also states of chronic, painless inflammation. Obesity, diabetes, allergies, asthma, and coronary heart disease are just a few examples of chronic inflammation.

Omega-3s are anti-inflammatory and pro-resolving. They increase circulation, enhance the immune system, and tell the body when to cease inflammatory cycles.

So, we need both of these fatty acids for optimal health,

even without concussion or brain trauma. Omega-6s and omega-3s really should be consumed in a balanced proportion. Mankind literally evolved over tens of thousands of years eating a diet balanced in omega-6s and omega-3s. Like omega-3s, omega-6s are also polyunsaturated fatty acids, but the chemical structure is different. They're not as flexible as omega-3s, but more importantly, the metabolites that derive from many omega-6s are very inflammatory.

The typical Western diet has changed so much over the last fifty to a hundred years that the ratios of omega-6s to omega-3s have become very imbalanced. If we're consuming way too many omega-6s, because of the typical Western diet, then our brains have become imbalanced in terms of omega-6s to omega-3s.

Our bodies are meant to be in balance, and this certainly holds true for omegas. With a 1:1 or 2:1 ratio of omega-6s to omega-3s, we would be protected. We could probably function very well if ratios were 4:1. We're meant to be relatively imbalanced because of the enzymatic processes, but not at the ratio we are currently.

So what is the average ratio of consumption? When I did a study with one of the leading psychiatrist researchers at the NIH looking at military suicide, we came up with a ratio of 25:1 in the military active-duty population. That's twenty-five units of inflammatory omega-6s for every unit of anti-inflammatory omega-3s.

Omega-6s are very pro-inflammatory and pro-thrombotic. This means the metabolites of omega-6s cause the blood to clot, and omega-3s balance or counter that process. Omega-3s are anti-inflammatory and anti-thrombotic and are there to balance the omega-6s so that the blood doesn't clot. That's part of the reason why omega-3s are so heart-healthy. That's why the Inuits demonstrated very little coronary heart disease—they were consuming very high levels of omega-3s.

Low levels of omega-3s lead to a significant influence on inflammation. When you have low omega-3 levels, you don't have the balance to offset the pro-inflammatory omega-6s, and you don't have an adequate ability to resolve the inflammation. This imbalance leads not only to increases in heart disease, but to increases in allergies, asthma, diabetes, and obesity. These are all very inflammatory diseases. By consuming less omega-3s and more omega-6s, we are changing the balance of the actual structure of our bodies to where we have less omega-3s and more omega-6s literally in our brains. Remember that omega-3s are actually "bricks of the brain"? Joseph Hibbeln, MD, my psychiatrist friend with the NIH, says, "Junk food equals junk brain," referring to the amount of omega-6s consumed by the typical American. I'm an optimist; I lean toward a more positive approach and say, "Healthy food equals a healthy brain."

While omega-3s are found in animal meat and fish, they are also related to what the animal eats. For example, grass-fed beef or field lamb are much higher in omega-3s than corn- and grain-fed beef because, remember, you are what you eat, and so are they. While people think chicken, for example, is a healthier meat choice, if you're feeding chicken corn and soybeans, which are high in omega-6s, you have chicken meat that is going to be high in omega-6s. The same holds true for farm-raised fish, tilapia being one of the worst in terms of too many omega-6s and almost no omega-3s.

So, although good sources of omega-3s are grass-fed beef and lamb, the best source is wild cold-water fatty fish, such as salmon, sardines, mackerel, and tuna. These fish are rich in DHA (docosahexaenoic acid), and EPA (eicosapentaenoic acid)—and remember, these are both types of omega-3 fatty acids. These oily fish can contain up to 30 percent oil, though this figure may vary. White fish, on the other hand, only contain high concentrations of oil in the liver, and their bodies have much less oil.

Interestingly enough, in the 1980s, NASA was trying to figure out how we could safely send astronauts on a three-year mission to Mars and back. They were working from the question: How do we provide nutrition to astronauts on a three-year mission where there is no access to fresh food? One of most important nutritional concerns was providing enough omega-3s. Somebody in that program asked the simple question, "Where do fish get their omega-3s?" The answer is they get it from eating the little fish that are eating algae. Then, of course, the food chain kicks in. The little fish get eaten by bigger fish, who then get eaten by bigger fish, and so on.

When NASA determined the omega-3s food chain began with algae, they developed a program to grow algae high in omega-3s which could be harvested in order to feed astronauts on a three-year mission to Mars. Then, in 1986, during spending cuts, the space program decided to nix the project. Fortunately, the scientists involved in the project felt their work was too important to let go, so they started their own company where they learned to grow algae in million-gallon tanks and extract the omega-3s directly. In this way the presence of mercury, heavy metals, PCBs, and toxins could be avoided because the algae is grown in a controlled environment without the risk of contamination from outside sources found in seafood.

In 2002, that company founded by NASA, Martek Biosciences (now owned by Royal DSM N.V.), began to get authorization and approval to put their algae-derived omega-3 DHA into infant formula. Today, almost 100 percent of all infant formula in the United States today is supplemented with clean, algae-derived DHA.

Why do most people have higher levels of omega-6s? The US diet has changed so much since World War II. You will hear me say this over and over again: You are what you eat...and so is the food chain. The biggest source of omega-6s in the American diet is from soybean oil. Remember, since the late 1960s soybean consumption has gone up astronomically. The McGovern Commission was conveyed from 1968 to 1977 to study hunger in America and looked at how to provide more calories to children. We had wiped out polio. We had put a man on the moon. Why did we still have starving children in Appalachia and different parts of the United States?

One of the pieces of legislation to come from the McGovern Commission was the Farm Bill. The Farm Bill was written into law as a means to subsidize farmers for producing the most calorically dense crops that are the easiest to grow. This translated into subsidies for soybean and corn. The amount of soybean that was grown and thus consumed in the United States immediately escalated exponentially. It just absolutely took off. Soybean is the biggest source of omega-6s. Why is that important? Because soybean oil is used in processed foods—so any food that's processed more than likely has omega-6s from soybean oil in it. Omega-6s are very shelf-stable. They don't spoil. You could leave a box of crackers out in the sun for a week, and they wouldn't spoil. Omega-3s are different—if you leave a fish out in the hot sun for an hour or two, it smells, well, like bad fish.

Subsequently, our food supply and the food chain have become saturated with soybean oil and omega-6s. Both the food supply and the food chain are imbalanced, and if you look at the impact on our brains, the effect reflects this imbalance. We have way too many omega-6s in our brain.

Trying to avoid omega-6s or reduce their consumption is one way to try and correct for this imbalance, but it is ineffective and almost impossible. Omega-6s are in everything—virtually every food in a box or package on the grocery shelf is laden with omega-6s. They are also not just in processed foods but in the animal feed that we use to fatten up our herds and flocks. Whether that's chicken, pork, or beef, all are fed soybean and corn which are high sources of omega-6s. These meats, in turn, become very high in omega-6s. Unfortunately, omega-3s remain terribly low in these animal food sources.

The second hurdle to just reducing omega-6s in our bodies is the fact that they are fats. Fats have a very long half-life, meaning they stay in our bodies for a very long time. Even if you could stop consuming or could cut back dramatically the omega-6s by eating really good grass-fed animal sources and no processed foods, it would still take a year or longer to decrease the levels of omega-6s in your body to a reasonable level. I am not diminishing the importance of omega-6s in our diet and the need to decrease them, but when faced with a brain injury or when seeking a preventive protocol, such a long-term solution is a luxury most people can ill afford. With brain trauma and concussion, time is critical. So to return to a balance between omega-6s and omega-3s, we need to work the other side of the equation. We need to increase the omega-3s—and this is something we can do immediately using The Omega-3 Protocol.

SIDE EFFECTS OF OMEGA-3S

The misconceptions surrounding the use of omega-3s vary from ill-informed to misinformed. I will keep it simple. There are no real side effects from taking omega-3s. The number-one misconception is that high doses of omega-3s may cause excess bleeding because it thins the blood, which is kind of silly. It is more accurate to say high doses of omega-3s decrease the ability for platelets to clot. But when I'm talking high doses that can affect bleeding, it really is upward of 40 grams or more a day, way more than almost anyone would ever take. Again, this is a balancing act. If you have a cut, you have to stop the bleeding, but if blood clots too much, then we have a medical issue. That's what a heart attack is—a blood clot forms, breaks off, and now we have an emergency. So, while it is biochemically plausible, high doses of omega-3s have never been shown in any clinical study to be an issue when it comes to bleeding or have been named as a source for uncontrolled bleeding. In fact, sometimes what you want is blood that will not clot easily.

An Italian study looked at success rates in coronary artery bypass surgery and the use of omega-3s. The researchers used one week of high doses of omega-3s prior to surgery and the patients not only had no problems with bleeding, but had improved outcomes and decreased numbers of days in the hospital and ICU, infections, and postsurgery depression. The head of general surgery at Oregon Health State University, Robert Martindale, MD, PhD, requires his patients to be on omega-3s for a week prior to any elective surgery. Dr. Martindale recently said on a webinar that we have to dispel this misperception that omega-3s cause bleeding. This comes from the guy who has a PhD in nutrition and writes the recommendations for the Society of Critical Care Medicine.

The biggest reason why they have these misconceptions is basically because when we entered the era of antibiotics and vaccines after World War II, medical schools ceased teaching nutrition because pharmaceuticals seemed to have many more answers. How do I put this? We're no longer a health-care system—we're a disease care system. Nutrition is vital for health but not considered important to treat disease. A large part of this mentality is because we're victims of our own successes. Though they produce important tools, the pharmaceutical, vaccine, and antibiotic industries have grown so powerful that the need to teach nutrition in medical schools has fallen by the wayside.

CAN WE MEASURE OMEGA-3S IN THE BLOOD?

In a word, yes. The only way to know your blood level of omega-3s is by measuring it. Most Americans have low levels of omega-3s in their blood. Omega-3s are important for heart, brain, and joint health and can be improved by simple dietary changes and/or supplementation. Whereas in the past, the decision to recommend omega-3 supplementation to a patient was rather subjective, the availability of tests to measure blood levels equips a physician with a tool to determine objectively whether or not to do so. Unfortunately, most physicians remain unaware that a blood test for omegas exists. This test can be done by most hospitals and major laboratory companies and may be covered by insurance.

I've found that the least expensive and most thorough way to test omega levels is direct-to-consumer testing. There are several at-home omega testing kits including OmegaQuant (omegaquant.com) and the Holman Bloodspot Test (lipidlab.com). Both labs provide the at-home test kit allowing individuals to supply a simple finger-prick sample of blood that can then be tested for a complete fatty-acid profile. The Holman Bloodspot Test is named for Dr. Ralph Holman, who invented the term "omega-3" and discovered the metabolism and definitive nature of omega-3s. Dr. Holman was the first person to measure omega-3s in the blood and his work lives on through his student and my good friend, Dr. Doug Bibus.

When you send in a bloodspot test to Dr. Bibus, you get a detailed report back that includes your Total Omega-3 Score, % Omega-3 HUFA, and Omega-3 Index, among other details. Your total Omega-3 Score is generated from the measured amount of omega-3s in your bloodstream, described as a percentage figure. For example, if your omega-3 score is 5 percent, it means that 5 percent of the total fatty acids in your blood are made up of omega-3s. In certain populations such as the Japanese, who consume large amounts of marine-based foods, the total omega-3 score is typically over 15 percent. That is a good goal for all of us.

The Omega-3 HUFA test also is known as the Lands' Test, named after Dr. Bill Lands who invented this test and terminology. Its technical name HUFA is an abbreviation for "highly unsaturated fatty acids." These fatty acids generally form the basis for our inflammatory response system. Dr. Lands established that a lower Omega-6 HUFA score with a higher Omega-3 HUFA score is the ideal condition and directly relates to low mortality rates from cardiovascular disease. Typical Americans have an Omega-3 HUFA score of 20 percent, which directly correlates to a high incidence of mortality from heart disease.

People having a score of 50 percent (balanced omega-3 and omega-6) correlates with an approximate 50 percent reduction in mortality. Populations having an Omega-3 HUFA score of 70 percent have a very low likelihood of cardiovascular mortality. I believe the same correlation exists when considering brain health.

The Omega-3 Index is the combined value of EPA and DHA. The science behind the Omega-3 Index resulted from the work of Siscovick and Albert, who examined omega-3 levels in populations and then assessed their risk of sudden death. According to Albert's data, increasing omega-3 blood values from 3.5 percent to 6.8 percent was correlated with a 90 percent reduction in risk of sudden cardiac death. Siscovick's work reported similar outcomes. The recommended Omega-3 Index is 8 percent or greater, meaning a combined percentage total of EPA and DHA greater than 8 percent.

Monitoring also is important. It's great to get a baseline test done to see where you are, but you should also retest again after about three months to see if the changes you made in eating habits or taking an omega-3 supplement are getting you to optimal levels. In a few cases, that might mean taking less fish oil on a daily basis, but that is the exception. Most people need more.

HOW DO OMEGA-3S HELP THE BRAIN TO HEAL?

The brain, like any other organ, needs nutritive support to

heal. To heal concussions, the consumption of omega-6s and omega-3s should be in balance. While it's important that we decrease the amount of omega-6s to help the body in the long-run, we need to increase the levels of omega-3s quickly to be able to help the brain heal. The two important omega-3s are EPA and DHA.

DHA is found in the brain and is an integral part of the cell membrane, comprising 30 percent of the dry weight of the brain. When broken down in the brain, DHA's downstream metabolites, have names like protectins and resolvins that describe exactly what they do. They help *protect* the brain from injury, and they help *resolve* inflammation when injury occurs.

While DHA is found in the brain, EPA is found in the blood vessels and our immune system. The downstream effect of the metabolites of EPA are called eicosanoids. Eicosanoids have a positive influence on inflammatory cells and decrease inflammation in the body. They also act to relax blood vessels, lowering blood pressure and allowing blood to flow deeper into the brain. When somebody has an injury and takes high doses of omega-3s, part of metabolic breakdown is the rush of EPA into the bloodstream. This rush allows blood to flow deeper into parts of the brain that may not have seen oxygen and nutrition on a regular basis, which is one of the reasons why people notice such an improvement so quickly.

In "Concussions, Traumatic Brain Injury, and the Innovative Use of Omega-3 Fatty Acids," an article featured in the *Journal of the American College of Nutrition*, I discuss how omega-3s offer the advantage of neuroprotection, control neuroinflammation, and help foster neuroregeneration. Patients may benefit from aggressively adding substantial amounts of omega-3s to optimize the nutritional foundation following TBI and concussion.

In another study funded by the NIH and published in the *Journal of Clinical Psychiatry* in 2011, we look at levels of omega-3s in suicide deaths. In 2009, I was doing some work with Joseph Hibbeln, MD, from the NIH. Dr. Hibbeln is a psychiatrist interested in how omega-3s help with mental health. One time, Dr. Hibbeln bemoaned the lack of evidence and jokingly mentioned that if we could just draw blood on people prior to committing suicide, we could answer a lot of questions.

I looked at him and said, "Well, that's easy." He looked at me like I was crazy, but I continued, "The US military has 45 million blood specimens sitting in a freezer in Silver Spring, Maryland, with all of the Department of Defense's data behind it. How many do you think we need?" We settled on eight hundred well-documented suicides confirmed by the Armed Forces Institute of Pathology that occurred in active-duty military between the beginning of 2002 and the end of 2008, focusing on the time when we were in Iraq and Afghanistan. We also looked at eight hundred well-matched controls to those suicides. In all,

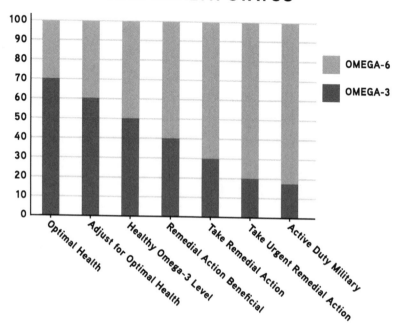

OMEGA-3 & OMEGA-6 LEVELS AND HEALTH STATUS

Legend: OMEGA-6, OMEGA-3

Categories: Optimal Health, Adjust for Optimal Health, Healthy Omega-3 Level, Remedial Action Beneficial, Take Remedial Action, Take Urgent Remedial Action, Active Duty Military Action

we were able to garner blood reports from those 1,600 people drawn within six months prior to the suicide deaths.

Our findings were twofold. First, we found the overall levels of omega-3s, DHA in particular, in the whole group were profoundly low among these US active-duty military personnel. The second finding was that these low levels of DHA correlated with a 62 percent increased risk in suicide.

That's pretty substantive. A 62 percent increase in risk of suicide was larger than any other mental-health indicator we could find, including if your best friend was killed in action right next to you. I presented this data to the US Army Surgeon General twice and he refused to believe it. Undaunted, we published it in the *Journal of Clinical Psychiatry*. Not long after, the story ran on the front page of *USA Today* and on *CNN Headline News*. The day after the story broke on *USA Today* and *CNN*, I was at a TBI conference where the keynote speaker was the Vice Chief of Staff of the Army, General Peter Chiarelli. After he walked off the stage, the press crowded around him asking questions about omega-3s, the brain, and suicide. As he was leaving, I stopped him and introduced myself as the person who published the study for which he was now having to answer. To his credit, he asked me to come to his office and teach him what he needed to know about omega-3s.

A week later on a Wednesday night in October 2011, I was in his office at the Pentagon showing General Chiarelli the science behind the story. It was just the two of us in his office plus his scientific advisor. I had warned the General that I was going to tell him the facts straight up and he wasn't going to like it. He agreed that was the best way. I half-jokingly told him I've been known to be trouble. After a few paper PowerPoint slides, General Chiarelli stopped me and asked, "Is this science or is this your opinion?"

I said, "No. This is other people's science. Here's the proof," pointing to the references at the bottom of each page. He looked at his scientific advisor, and she nodded her head yes.

I understood his hesitancy when he asked, "Well. What's the downside?"

I said, "What do you mean downside? There is no downside. It's just fish oil. It's nutrition."

General Chiarelli cocked his head said, "That's not what the Army Surgeon General tells me."

"Well, what does he tell you?" I was genuinely curious.

"Well, he said there can be side effects if you take too much and..."

I didn't catch the last bit of his sentence because I started laughing.

"What's so funny?"

"He's full of BS," somehow slipped out of my mouth before I could stop it. I don't know why I felt so emboldened. Maybe because I knew I was right.

The General paused for a moment. "Wait a minute. You're telling me that the US Army Surgeon General, Lieutenant General Schumacher, an MD and PhD from Harvard Medical School is full of BS?"

"Yes, sir. That's what I'm telling you." Then I thought a moment. "Let me prove it to you." I pulled a bottle of fish oil out of my pocket, and I put it down in front of him on his desk. He said he already takes fish oil. "How much?" I asked.

"One or two every morning."

"Here's what you're going to do. You're to take the same dose I use in The Omega-3 Protocol, the same dose I would put a nineteen-year-old private on if he had an exposure to an improvised explosive device (IED) explosion and was having concussive symptoms. You're going to take five capsules starting tomorrow morning with breakfast. Five with lunch. Five with dinner. Fifteen capsules a day just for the next two days. There's only thirty capsules in here, so you're set. I promise you won't have any side effects and you will notice a difference."

We wrapped up as he needed to get to a dinner. As he flew down the hall, he yelled back toward me over his right shoulder, "Doc, you and I are going to be best friends!" And then he disappeared. His scientific advisor just looked at me, shook her head, and said, "Strap on your seatbelt. It's going to be a wild ride."

Three days later on Saturday morning, I had an email from the scientific advisor. General Chiarelli was on his way down to Pentagon City to buy more fish oil. What should he get? I had my own questions to ask. Did he have any side effects? Answer: No. Did he notice any difference? The answer that came back made me laugh again. "Yes. That's why he's going to buy more fish oil."

And then she continued, "Not only did he notice a difference, but his staff noticed a difference, and most importantly, his wife noticed a difference."

This bode well. I thought Joe Hibbeln and I were

moving toward preventing suicide among service men and women. And then...nothing happened.

When General Chiarelli retired a number of months later, I called him on his personal cell phone and asked him what had happened—why weren't we moving forward introducing omega-3s into the diets of service men and women? The General sighed. "I let happen exactly what you told me not to let happen. The Medical Corps threw science in the way as roadblocks saying there was no evidence that it would work, so instead they would rather do nothing." In short, nothing changed in the diets of the military and there was no nutritional support offered to service personnel. Sad, but true, the military would rather have done nothing than try something as simple as nutrition. Meanwhile, one active-duty military person continued to commit suicide every thirty-six hours.

Eventually, the Army decided to actually launch a study and offer funds to the NIH and Joe Hibbeln to conduct a randomized, placebo-controlled, clinical trial. They've spent around twelve million dollars, struggled with enrollment, and have only looked at veterans in the VA hospital in Charleston, South Carolina, and they won't achieve their intended outcomes. From my point of view, they've wasted twelve million dollars paying people to try to do a study. Twelve million dollars can buy a lot of fish oil, and the Army could be making an immediate difference in people's lives.

The American Psychiatric Association recommends people consume at least two grams of omega-3s a day. This was based on studies going back as far as 1996 looking at omega-3s and bipolar disorder and depression. This last recommendation came out in 2011. As far as I am concerned, that represents two grams of fish oil almost no one ever takes.

GRASSROOTS RESEARCH AND EDUCATION

The cost of studies with clinical trials and control groups, peer review, and replication is prohibitively high. These studies cost millions of dollars and take years to complete. No pharmaceutical company is interested in wanting to fund such a study because you can get fish oil at your local grocery store. With little to no financial incentive for companies to do such a study, research remains a result of dogged determination and a passion for the subject. Julian Bailes and I remain at the foci of most research, and the Brain Health Education and Research Institute remains the mecca for the education about omega-3s, concussion, and TBI.

Research is a top-down approach. At the Brain Health Education and Research Institute, I try to help guide and participate in research in this area and a position I am comfortable with. Shifting findings beyond the medical literature, however, is a different process. How do you change how medicine is practiced? I also wanted to take the education route, a more grassroots approach, but one that can be very powerful. How do I reach you, the parent, coach, or doctor?

How do I get *you* to think about fish oil?

This is the grassroots approach. How do you change America? Moms. Moms can change America. "Soccer moms" need to think about using fish oil proactively so their kids are healthier and their brains can withstand a shock without instantly becoming inflamed. I assert we can protect the brain by proactively feeding it omega-3s and eating healthy. And I make this assertion by looking at associated studies.

Since there are no direct studies in humans about using omega-3s to protect the brain from injury, I looked into animal studies. Julian Bailes published several on traumatic brain injury using omega-3s. In three related studies, Bailes looked at when rats were fed omega-3s, after and before trauma. In all the studies, rats were concussed. In the first study they were fed omega-3s for thirty days after the injury. Those fed omega-3s had a significantly better recovery than those who were not fed the fatty acids. He replicated the study using just DHA and had similar findings.

The third study looked at nutritional support before injury. In this study, rats were fed DHA thirty days prior to concussion. All injuries were made with the same level of concussion causing pressure against the skull. In the

DHA-fed group, either injuries were not noticeable or the rats appeared injury-free. In the control groups, concussion was assessed in all rats, and recovery was along the timeline expected.

Studies led by the group working for Nick Bazan, MD, PhD, at Louisiana State University New Orleans, NeuroScience Center, looked at using DHA in experimental stroke animal models. These studies have found huge improvements or protection using DHA, either when the stroke was temporarily induced for just 30 minutes or a permanent stroke.

Professor Adina Michael-Titus, a researcher at the University of London, has had a profound impact on my work, and we have become good friends as well. She works on spinal cord injuries. What she found is if DHA is given to animals within three hours of a spinal cord injury, the animals maintain or retain their ability to walk. If DHA is given after three hours or not at all, that locomotive ability is lost. She also compared these outcomes with tissue samples from placebos, which is how she could make the claim that omega-3s help heal spinal cord injury. But she went even further. Michael-Titus ran a comparison and gave arachidonic acid omega-6s as supplementation after injury. The amount of damage the spinal cord undergoes when the system was flooded with omega-6s proved devastating. Basically, the injury was exacerbated.

DHA REDUCES PROGRESSION OF SPINAL CORD INJURY

Intravenous administration 1-hour after injury

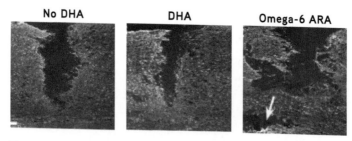

The spinal cord was surgically cut. This is what the spinal cord looks like after a week. The DHA group not only had less anatomic defect but also better locomotive outcome measures. The omega-6 group had a profoundly worse outcome with a huge amount of secondary damage in addition to the surgical injury.

SOURCE King, et al., J. Neurosci. 2006, 26,4672-4680.

One of Joe Hibbeln's colleagues at the NIH, Dr. Hee-Yong Kim, has shown that DHA helps neurons grow and improves the synaptic connections between neurons. This means that omega-3s would have a direct impact on patients by regrowing neurons and neuron connections (synapses) after an injury or illness.

By looking at the myriad of studies proving the importance of omega-3s in other aspects of brain and neurological injury and recovery, we can make the claim that omega-3s could be taken as a preventive. As you will see, I am not the only one who thinks this, and coaches across the country are paying attention and asking their athletes to take fish oil.

Okay. So this hits home. Not long after I started looking into the benefits of fish oil and omega-3s, my younger brother, Jamie, called me. He was at a Durham Bulls game, a minor-league baseball team in North Carolina. At some point during the game, they had a sumo wrestling contest, in which Jamie decided he needed to participate. As it turned out, he could not sumo wrestle a sumo wrestler and he subsequently got slammed to the ground—knocked unconscious.

Jamie called later that day and told me the whole story. You can imagine what I told him to take.

He said, "I already take fish oil because you hammered that into me."

I remained unmoved. "Then take more."

"You're kidding."

I was not.

"How much?"

"Why don't you take five capsules now and five before you go to bed? Then five the next morning and three times a day for the next week." That's pretty much how I came up with The Omega Protocol. By coincidence, it turns out that the five-capsule dose, which provides 3,000 milligrams of combined EPA and DHA, works out to be 40 milligrams per kilogram, the exact dose Julian Bailes fed the rats in his studies. This protocol has become what I routinely offer patients.

Ten years before, my brother had a stroke as a result of a pharmaceutical medication he was prescribed. Luckily, he fully recovered from the stroke and went on with his life. But he also struggled with depression. So although the exchange above is related in a relatively lighthearted way, there was some real concern. The next afternoon he called again, but he was not just reporting on his symptoms of concussion. He proceeded to tell me he had stopped taking his antidepressant medications about six months before and could feel himself spiraling downward. I listened, concerned, perhaps, that this could eventually lead to debilitating depression and suicide.

There was a pause, and then Jamie explained how, after just a day and half on fish oil, he felt better, more engaged. I listened and will never forget his words: "I don't know how to tell you this, but I'll just say that I feel a profound sense of happiness I've not felt in a long time."

He still takes five capsules of fish oil a day—and no antidepressants. Pharmaceuticals almost killed him, but fish oil keeps him much healthier today.

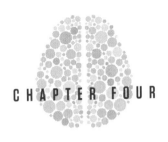

CHAPTER FOUR

HEAD TO HEAD— TRAUMATIC BRAIN INJURY

SOCCER HEADS

My son used to play soccer with a very competitive club up through eighth grade. When he was on the U13 team, he played alongside the most gifted player on the team, the coach's son. The father had played on the Gambia men's national team for four years starting when he was in high school, at just sixteen. When he was twenty, his family immigrated to the United States. Now, his son, Tamani, is being groomed for the US Junior Olympic team and is listed as one of the top one hundred IMG players to watch. He will graduate in 2018, no doubt with scholarship offers flooding his mailbox.

At a high-level game, Tamani collided with another player. Now we are talking about the top-ranking players in the league, in the nation. They play hard and fast, and it is very, very, physical. I didn't see the game or the injury since it was when Tamani was playing on a different team for that game. He was out for a couple weeks with a concussion. I found out because I asked my son where Tamani had disappeared to, and he said, "Apparently, he had a concussion and he can't play for a couple weeks." Tamani was totally out of the picture.

The father coached eight different teams and catching up with him was hard. Finally, one time, the father showed up for our game and I asked him about Tamani. He sighed and said his son was still really having difficulty recovering. He continued to suffer from headaches, seemed withdrawn, slept a lot, and had zero concentration. With all these symptoms, Tamani was unable to attend school and was getting far behind.

I told him about The Omega Protocol and explained how he should get Tamani started on high doses of fish oil right away. The very next weekend, Tamani showed up for the game. Both his parents were there and Tamani was ready to play. His mother sought me out right before the kickoff. She went on to talk about how the headaches went away almost immediately, that the gregarious, wrestling play between her two sons had returned, that Tamani could concentrate on schoolwork enough to catch up in all his classes, and that his personality seemed restored. Tamani was now the outgoing kid he always had been. She closed her story by giving me a big hug, and said, "Basically, thank you. You gave us our son back."

CONCUSSION 101: THE BASICS

Now, we're going to delve into the science of concussion, but I have to keep it simple enough that even I can understand it! Basically, when somebody has a concussion, it is the result of a violent shaking of the brain or a transfer of mechanical energy to the brain. The violent shaking could be from falling and striking the head. It could be from heads colliding, getting an elbow to the head, running into a cement wall on a badly designed basketball court, or a myriad of other obstacles and events. The transfer of mechanical energy could be from a bomb or the close proximity of an IED to a soldier in a war zone where the blast wave goes through the brain.

The result is the same, however. Concussion, in its most simple terms, is a bruising of the brain. Inside the skull, the brain is bathed in cerebrospinal fluid to cushion it and offer some protection. When the head gets shaken violently or energy gets transmitted through the brain, the cushioning effect is not enough to prevent injury, so the brain hits the inside of the skull and the brain is bruised. Even if you're wearing a helmet, the brain still gets bounced around inside the skull.

When the brain slams up against the skull and is bruised, that is what we call the primary injury and concussion. It is an example of the power of inertia. If you've got this gelatinous mass moving inside the skull at a constant speed and the head suddenly stops, like in a car accident, the inertia of the brain keeps it moving forward until it strikes the inside of the skull.

Think of an egg. If you shake an egg, the yolk is going to hit up inside the shell. Better, think of a bowl of jelly. If you slide the bowl quickly, the jelly slaps the side of the bowl. Common sports concussions are the coup-contre-coup injuries. If somebody hits their head, forehead to forehead for example, the brain bounces forward, hits the front of the skull (coup) and then reverberates and bounces back, hitting the back of the skull (contracoup). You can actually get a double bruising, one on the coup or the front side of the brain, and the second on the contrecoup, or the back side of the brain.

What many people don't realize is that the brain is not just one density like egg yolk or jelly. The brain actually has many different structures with many different densities, which all move at different speeds. Newton's first law of motion states that a body at rest will stay at rest until a net external force acts upon it and that a body in motion will remain in motion at a constant velocity until acted on by a net external force. That outside force may be a sudden deceleration, such as if you're going sixty miles an hour and you hit a cement wall and come to a very quick stop. In that scenario, your brain was traveling at sixty miles an hour, and it continues to travel at that speed and stops at a different rate as hits the inside of the skull. The substructures of the brain are of different densities. This means the different parts of the brain can move at different rates or stop at different rates. The result is what is called "shearing" of the connections between those different parts of the brain. It is this shearing and tearing of the fine tissues of the brain that result in many symptoms of a more severe TBI or a really bad concussion. This is what we call a diffused axonal injury (DAI).

Both types of injury are called primary injuries. The secondary injuries are a result of biochemical cascades that can occur. These involve an array of cellular processes. The primary injury, when somebody goes to the emergency room, often results in a CT scan (computerized tomography scan). Basically, a CT scan for a head injury is essentially only a decision-making tool to determine the need for emergency surgery. The physicians are looking for bleeding inside the skull. DAI will not appear on a CT scan. Doctors are not going to see the bruising on the brain with the CT scan used in the emergency room.

Starting immediately after the initial injury, the secondary injury begins. A biochemical cascade follows at the cellular level.

The primary injury sets off inflammatory and cellular cascades that start right after the primary injury and can last for seconds, minutes, hours, days, even weeks or months following the initial injury. This is why sometimes a patient can linger for two weeks or more, and their health continues to deteriorate along with their prognosis. Sometimes patients can feel and act fine, and all of the sudden, a week or a few weeks later, they start to have issues. There is compelling research demonstrating that all these different biochemical, inflammatory cascades continue over time.

A biochemical cascade is what happens whenever there is an injury. If you careen around your kitchen table and slam a hip into the corner, you may get some inflammation. The inflammation in that hip is quite necessary. It brings the proper nutrients and hormonal signals to help that injured area heal. The problem is, if that inflammation is out of control and continues on an inflammatory path, this creates a cascade of inflammation. Here's where the omega-6s and omega-3s come into play. If our bodies are imbalanced between the omega-6s and the omega-3s, that inflammatory process flares out of control and doesn't get resolved by the anti-inflammatory.

Think of a house fire. Imagine the fire department arrives and puts out the fire, yet it continues to smolder. Like inflammation, this fire could continue to smolder and smolder and smolder and may burst back into flames,

CONTINUED DAMAGE FOLLOWING INITIAL INJURY

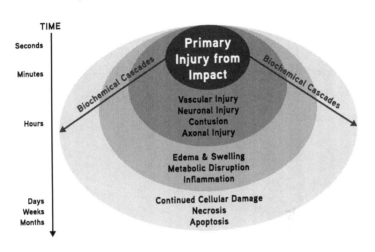

or it may just continue to slowly burn through the house and destroy everything. Inflammation will continue to destroy neurons and the cells of the brain unless that inflammation is brought under control. Given our diets and the imbalance of our omega-3s and omega-6s as typical Americans, that inflammation doesn't get under control as well, or as quickly, as it should. Adding omega-3s is like dousing the flames of inflammation.

In the brain, like in the hip, inflammation occurs after injury. There is often edema, or swelling of the brain. Edema is extracellular, which simply means "outside the cells" where the contents of cells have been released. There might be bleeding as well. Then there are the cells themselves that are affected. A cascade results from an influx of calcium and changes in calcium, sodium, potassium, and glutamate levels to where these four elements are flowing in and out of the cells at a rate not viable to keep the injured cells alive. The cells will eventually die off over the next couple of minutes to hours to days, or even weeks.

FEED A COLD...AND A COMA

It used to be the medical profession's edict, "Well, they're in a coma, so their metabolic needs are not great," because the patient appeared to be in a resting state. What researchers have found, after a mild concussion or severe TBI with coma, is the metabolic needs of the brain are actually dramatically increased. The greater the injury, the greater the metabolic needs are increased.

Your metabolic basal rate is almost doubled when you have a head injury. The brain consumes a vast percentage of calories every day, and when injured, it consumes even more. The brain consumes more energy to heal itself and to deal with all the biochemical changes occurring at the site of injury.

At Cornell University, Dr. Roger Härtl studied mortality rates and nutritional support at four and seven days after brain injury. In their 2008 article "Effective Early Nutrition on Deaths Due to Severe Traumatic Brain Injury" in the *Journal of Neurosurgery*, Härtl and three other authors reported that patients who were not fed within four and seven days after a TBI had a two- and fourfold increase in likelihood of death, respectively. In fact, when somebody is in a coma from a concussion, we now know nutritional support is paramount to recovery.

Clearly, if you don't feed the brain the proper nutrition, it can't heal. Sodium and potassium in an IV may keep a patient hydrated, but salt water is not nutrition. Often, patients in a coma receive no nutritional support at all or, at the very least, just some basic slurry of processed liquid. If a patient is not provided actual, nutritional food, and this starvation persists for a week, Härtl proved that week would see a fourfold increase in risk of death.

If there's any doubt as to why I started the Brain Health Education and Research Institute or any question about the need to change how modern medicine is practiced when it comes to TBI and concussions, this kind of research will give proof that they are necessary. The state of our medical system and how we approach TBI and concussion appalls me sometimes, and it should appall you as well. I hope that we can get doctors and nurses in the medical system to remember that nutrition is vital to life and healing. Seems kinda basic, doesn't it? I thought so, too.

SYMPTOMS AND MISCONCEPTIONS OF CONCUSSION

When a person suffers a bump, blow, or jolt to the head or

body, he or she is at risk of having a concussion or more serious brain injury. There is a subtle difference between signs and symptoms. Signs are what a doctor, parent, coach, or another person observes about the person injured. Possible signs observed in a person who may have had a concussion include the following:

- The person can't recall events prior to or after a hit or fall.
- The person appears dazed, stunned, or confused.
- The person moves clumsily or is unable to maintain his or her balance.
- The person repeats questions or answers questions slowly.
- The person loses consciousness (even just for a moment).
- The person shows mood, behavior, or personality changes.

Symptoms are what a person reports he or she is experiencing. According to the CDC, the symptoms of concussion usually fall into four broad categories: (1) Physical, (2) Cognitive, (3) Emotional, and (4) Sleep. The one most patients report, however, is "brain fog," a non-medical term that is still very appropriate and descriptive.

Physical symptoms include headache or "pressure" in the head, nausea or vomiting, balance problems or dizziness, blurry or double vision, sensitivity to light and noise, numbness or tingling, and just an overall sense of not "feeling right."

Cognitive symptoms can include difficulty thinking clearly, trouble concentrating, difficulty remembering, feeling slowed down, or feeling sluggish, hazy, foggy, or groggy.

Emotional symptoms are those of irritability, sadness or depression, anxiety or nervousness, or just being in an overly emotional state.

Sleep-related symptoms are a really big issue following concussions. Patients can be fatigued as a result of disturbed sleeping patterns. Their energy level typically is low, and they tire easily. Getting through the day may seem Herculean. I've dealt with some NFL players who are exhausted by noon. This is all a result of prior brain trauma. One time just a few years ago, I met up with a television personality, a retired NFL player, at 9:00 on a Monday morning. We did an hour taping for a television show, had lunch, and returned to his house. Then he excused himself by explaining, "I'm exhausted; I need to take a nap. Mondays are just murder. They're just so strenuous." His energy level was zero.

And then there's brain fog. Think of when you've had a bad head cold and it felt as if your head was stuffed with cotton. Remember how difficult it was to think clearly? Or how your energy felt constantly sapped until the cold went away? Now imagine that feeling all the time without the runny nose, coughing, and sneezing. That's what brain fog is like after a concussion.

In my practice, working with both children and adults, the most common symptoms are headaches, brain fog,

SYMPTOMS OF CONCUSSION USUALLY FALL INTO FOUR CATEGORIES:

Thinking/ Remembering	Physical	Emotional/ Mood	Sleep
Difficulty thinking clearly	Headache Fuzzy or blurry vision	Irritability	Sleeping more than usual
Feeling slowed down	Nausea or vomiting (early on) Dizziness	Sadness	Sleep less than usual
Difficulty concentrating	Sensitivity to noise or light Balance problems	More emotional	Trouble falling asleep
Difficulty remembering new information	Feeling tired, having no energy	Nervousness or anxiety	

SOURCE http://www.cdc.gov/traumaticbraininjury/symptoms.html

fatigue, just having no energy, personality and mood changes, and irritability. People, both adults and children, can become much more irritable than usual. Sometimes, that's difficult to see in a teenager. How do you know when a teenager is more irritable? You have to be the judge and jury. When in doubt, ask them questions: Did you fall? Did you hit your head? What else are you feeling? Teens in particular often tend to withdraw.

One misconception is that symptoms only appear the day of the injury. Symptoms can show up immediately if the injury is significant enough, but sometimes symptoms may not be readily apparent for days or even a couple weeks. Say your son or daughter has a concussion playing soccer in August, and there are two or three more weeks before school starts. Everything seems fine until mental stress coincides with the start of school. Now, irritability, brain fog, and fatigue all set in and are unmasked with the added stress of school. Concussion is involved.

The other misconception is that concussion only results when consciousness is lost. This is simply not true. This is critical: you don't have to be knocked unconscious to have a concussion. In fact, the overwhelming majority of concussions don't involve being knocked unconscious.

About three years ago, one of my West Point classmates was the Commandant of Cadets, as a one-star, Brigadier General. As a result of conversations with him, he asked me to come up to West Point and review how the US Military Academy handled concussions.

I went to New York several times over the following couple of months and evaluated a system that proved to be almost nonexistent. I made a number of recommendations about how they could create a concussion program. One major recommendation was that the concussion program, including baseline neurocognitive testing, needed to be expanded to the entire Corps of Cadets, not just the Division I collision-sport athletes. Later that year, the General was at a meeting in Washington, DC. I met up with him and he told me the program was already paying dividends.

For example, they had a cadet who was academically at the top of his class after his freshman year at West Point. He was also on the intercollegiate wrestling team. In his sophomore year, he suddenly began failing classes. You don't go from being number one in your class at West Point to failing. They brought him into the concussion program, performed some of the testing I recommended, and realized he was not functioning at the level he should have been. He was, essentially, brain damaged; his neurocognitive functioning was significantly impaired. When they really researched and did more testing, they determined he had suffered a couple of concussions all without losing consciousness. They were able to pull him out of classes and send him home to rest for the remainder of the school year. When he returned and repeated his sophomore year, he had recovered, and so did his performance in the classroom.

This also reminds me to say a few words here about academics. All the attention is placed on sports and Return-to-Play protocols regarding how fast we can get an athlete back to playing a game. Personally, I think we need to be paying much greater attention to Return-to-Learn or Return-to-Academics. Sports and outdoor activities are great, and I'm a huge fan of playing hard, but there is no substitute in life for a good academic education unimpaired by a concussion that doesn't fully recover.

SCORE CARD: CONCUSSION IN THE UNITED STATES

According to the CDC, in 2010 there were about 2.5 million emergency room visits, hospitalizations, or deaths associated with traumatic brain injury in the United States. The number of unreported concussions keeps escalating. The CDC once claimed that there were 1.7 million brain injuries annually. Now, they have shifted the needle to three or four million. Their rationale is that for each reported case, there is at least another one or two that are unreported.

The standard treatment, according to the CDC, is to rest, take it slow, and talk to your health-care provider. Patients and parents are encouraged to provide cognitive and physical rest, meaning no physical exertion and no screen time, no computers, no television, and no electronics for up to two weeks. They want patients to go sit in a dark room for fourteen days. You can imagine telling your teenage son or daughter this delightful news. And there are no nutritional guidelines at all, whether from the CDC or NIH or any government agency out there. There is literally no discussion about nutrition and how nutrition could help recovery from concussion.

Basically, that has been the standard treatment: physical and cognitive rest with no studying, no electronics, and no exercise for up to two weeks until symptoms are completely cleared. Go sit in a dark closet for two weeks, and hopefully you will get better. A few years ago, I was in Germany for a meeting about the intravenous omega-3 formulation I mentioned before. After a long day of meetings and discussion, I was in a pub having a beer with Professor Adina Michael-Titus, the world-renowned spinal cord injury researcher and friend of mine who was hoping she would be able to use my product for spinal cord injury patients. I was lamenting that we didn't seem to be doing anything different for TBI from what we did 500 years ago. She said, "Oh, that's not true. It's been at least a thousand!"

Thankfully, this is starting to change. For example, Dr. Jamshid Ghajar, Director of the Stanford University Concussion and Brain Performance Center, Clinical Professor of Neurosurgery, and the founder of the Brain Trauma Foundation, works with athletes and concussion. At the concussion clinic at Stanford, they put athletes on the treadmill the day after they have a concussion because they have come to believe exercise is critical to healing. What he and his team are finding is, just like after a knee or back injury, the patient might need a day or two of rest but then needs to rally and exercise.

New research suggests those who exercise within a week of injury, regardless of symptoms, have nearly half as many concussion symptoms that linger more than a month than those who do not exercise in this time frame. Dr. Roger Zemek in Ottawa, reporting on a study he recently completed of over three thousand child concussions, says, "Exercise within seven days of injury was associated with nearly half the rate of persistent post-concussive symptoms, or those that last beyond a month."

CDC is woefully behind, in part because the research is moving so fast. But the individual health-care providers and concussion clinics at major university athletic programs are realizing that high-level athletes can't sit around doing nothing for two weeks. They have to at least be exercising. There is good reason to make sure there is adequate blood flow to the brain for recovery. This is just part of aging and good health. One of the most compelling reasons for regular exercise is to have good, consistent blood flow to the brain, and that's achieved principally through exercise.

After a head injury, you want to have good blood flow to the brain. Therefore, patients need to exercise. But exercise should not be to the point of having worsening or additional symptoms, and should never put the patient's head at risk of another concussion. Recent research on subsymptom threshold exercise (SSTE) demonstrates higher rates of healing when exercise is incorporated into a strategy for recovery. SSTE is based on heart rate. The heart rate is calculated at the point the patient starts to have symptoms, and then the patient holds exercise exertion to 80 percent of that heart rate for two weeks. After two weeks, the athlete should go to maximum exercise tolerance and see if the symptoms return, and if so, determine at what heart rate and then readjust the SSTE for another two weeks. One study showed that the exercise actually changed patients' brains from abnormal to normal. According to Dr. John Leddy at the University of Buffalo, "It changed the blood flow in their brain from an abnormal pattern that we saw with concussion to a normal pattern that we saw with healthy people. In this case we are hoping that by engaging the beneficial effects of exercise and the physiology of the brain, that this will actually speed recovery in kids with acute concussion."

STROKE AND CONCUSSION

The difference between a stroke and a concussion is in primary cause. A stroke is either a blood clot or a bleed in the brain that deprives the brain of blood flow and subsequently oxygen and nutrition. When that happens, those biochemical cascades, those secondary injuries, start to occur just as in concussion.

Concussion and traumatic brain injury is the result of physical injury, a physical transfer of mechanical energy to the brain or a part of the brain or through the whole brain. A stroke would be considered an acquired brain injury rather than a traumatic brain injury.

Because the trajectories for that biochemical cascade are similar to those for TBI, stroke studies are also important to look at when developing TBI treatment protocols. All the research going into traumatic and acquired brain injuries focus on what interventions can be used to modulate a secondary injury and to calm those biochemical cascades. If we can decrease the amount of cell death that occurs after the initial injury and stop those biochemical cascades, patients will recover faster and, perhaps, with less lingering effects.

This is, again, where omega-3s address the secondary injury. Neuroprotection helps with neuroinflammation and neuroregeneration. No drug currently addresses this trifecta of healing. If there's not enough neuroprotection to save brain cells from the continuing burning of neuroinflammation, then more cells are going to continue to die and be destroyed, and neurogeneration will not take place. If left untreated, the biochemical cascade will continue to destroy more and more brain tissue, unless brought under control, and that's the job of omega-3s and other antioxidants.

Inflammation is important after an injury, but it needs to be balanced and resolved. What omega-3s do is help regulate that inflammation and balance it so the brain can heal. Below is a really simple graphic demonstrating inflammation and the reaction to the inflammation and what happens when omega-3s are introduced.

SYSTEMIC INFLAMMATORY RESPONSE AND COMPENSATORY ANTI-INFLAMMATORY RESPONSE AS A CONSEQUENCE OF A MAJOR INSULT, AND THE MODULATING INFLAMMATORY HOMEOSTASIS-MAINTAINING EFFECT OF A BALANCED N-3 : N-6 RATIO

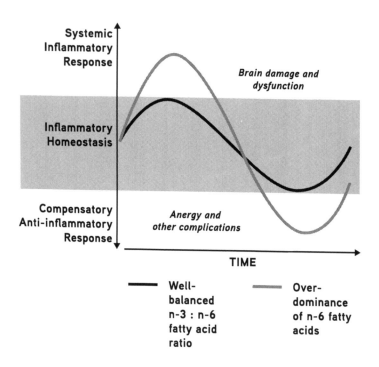

BART'S STORY

In 2000, when Bart Goldstein was sixteen, he was in a severe car accident in Upstate New York and then flown to Westchester County Medical Center. *No Stone Unturned: A Father's Memoir of His Son's Encounter with Traumatic*

Brain Injury is a book penned by his father, Joel Goldstein, detailing the process the whole family underwent through Bart's accident and rehabilitation. It's a wonderful book about how traumatic brain injury impacts the entire family, not just the patient. As Joel describes in his book:

Conventional medicine only takes survivors of severe TBI so far, often ending at the nursing home door, or heavily medicated at home, facing long empty hours and overwhelming family resources. Unconventional therapies are not merely a reasonable option, they're a necessity... After a month-long coma, Bart gradually emerged with crippling cognitive, emotional and physical deficits. After eight months of grueling hospital therapies, the school district and the hospital agreed he was not ready to return to class and would be better served by being placed in an institution. Out of desperation, we railed against warehousing our sixteen-year-old son in a convalescent home and fought time and time again for a chance for Bart to struggle, heal, and make progress.

I reached out to Joel Goldstein when I read an article authored by him on the *BrainLine* website and discovered that while Bart had been taking nutritional supplements recommended by some of his health-care providers, his regime included little omega-3s. I convinced Joel he should try The Omega Protocol and put Bart on high doses of fish oil. Bart had been in a coma for months after the accident, but now it was twelve years after the accident. Could fish oil make any improvement? In an email last year, Joel shared, "Bart has been on the high dose protocol for four months now and has continued cumulative improvements in short term memory, impulse control and now recently, fine motor control. We're delighted, and not really expecting to see, such global improvements twelve years post-accident." Then in a different email he reported Bart had improved fine-motor control so well that he had recently taken up playing the guitar.

Even more excited, Joel chatted with me on the phone late one night. He told me that the family joined Bart for dinner at a Korean restaurant, and Bart, without saying a word, picked up chopsticks with his damaged right hand and proceeded to eat dinner, even picking up single grains of rice. The family sat there completely dumbfounded at this newly reacquired skill. Previously, Bart had been told at occupational therapy that he would only ever have 15 percent functionality of his right hand.

That the introduction of omega-3s into the diet of a young man with TBI can have observable, positive effects twelve years after the initial injury speaks to the amazing healing power of the brain. More and more, neuroscientists and other researchers are discovering how plastic the brain really is, and the ability to grow and heal is greater than we thought. Nutrition helps provide a more neuro-permissive environment that supports brain healing.

CHAPTER FIVE

THE OMEGA PROTOCOL FOR CONCUSSION

DR. BILL

Dr. Bill Sears, otherwise known as "Dr. Bill," is a pediatrician and author in the Los Angeles area who is both well-known and well-respected, with over forty-five books published on pediatric health and wellness, including a book in 2012 titled *The Omega-3 Effect*. He has been referenced on the cover of *TIME Magazine*, has appeared on national television and radio, and has been published in both popular magazines and scientific journals. In November 2014, while on a medical mission in Kingston, Jamaica, he suffered a blow to his head and a pretty significant concussion. Even into the following months after the initial injury, he found himself still suffering with symptoms of concussion, the result of secondary trauma and the effects of biochemical cascades.

I met up with Dr. Sears for lunch at his house the following February, nearly four months after his initial injury. Though mostly recovered, he was still suffering from some headaches and brain fog. While in Jamaica, he had stood up suddenly and was struck in the head with a piece of medical equipment. His concussion was not severe, but he couldn't shake the symptoms. We were colleagues and friends. I knew he was incredibly health-conscious, and even though he was already taking omega-3s, I convinced him to take more. The amount of omega-3s he was taking wasn't enough and he needed to up his dosage. I pushed for The Omega Protocol. Dr. Sears agreed and he started that afternoon. Within a week, all symptoms resolved. His headaches vanished, and his brain fog lifted.

What was happening, of course, was that the biochemical cascades were being doused with fish oil and so the inflammation was turning off. The fuel feeding those pro-inflammatory biochemical cascades, omega-6s, were now in balance with the resolving power of the omega-3s, resulting in a reduction of inflammation. Once that reduction took place, Dr. Sears' symptoms resolved. With nutritional support, his brain healed itself.

I like facts. Once researched, tested, proven, and presented, facts allow better decisions to be made. I had asked a question, "What could I do?" for troops returning with TBI, and that question served as a catalyst for putting together a research study. When I started talking about the purpose of the study, the scientific communication grapevine proved strong, and I gathered up potential patients as it grew. People started contacting me, asking questions like, "What should I do? My father/brother/son/daughter has suffered a concussion. Should they take fish oil? How much? What kind? How soon will they improve?"

What I discovered is that, while surgical interventions following acute traumatic brain injury have been greatly advanced by military neurosurgeons and neurocritical care specialists in the past decade, medical treatment after the acute, life-saving phase of brain injury remains unchanged over the last century. This approach clearly needs to change. We know omega-3 fatty acids are the foundation of the neuron cell membrane, those "bricks of the brain." What new research keeps pointing to is the clear fact that providing nutritional foundation in therapeutic doses following injury provides the opportunity for healing and neuroregeneration of the brain. Our brains need a "neuropermissive" environment to heal.

This initial wave of my research, data gathering, and contact with others in the field and patients, began to surge in 2008. Right about that time was when my brother called me with his failed sumo wrestling story. I wrote down the protocol I gave him in a Word document so I could copy and paste the information into emails. It made answering questions less time-consuming and I could reach out to more patients and families. Over time, and with further research, dosages and durations became linked to, and dependent on, the type and extent of the initial injury and each patient's history.

Daily routines of adding fish oil to the diet for maintenance and nutrition turn out to be different than postconcussion dosages and are often a matter of nomenclature. Dosages also need to be to be much higher when treating severe TBI. The most accurate approaches to treatment use the actual omega-3 fatty acid names, EPA plus DHA, rather than "fish oil," and it is the amounts of those fatty acids we must adhere to in nutritional treatment plans.

The FDA's Generally Recognized as Safe, or GRAS, dosage is 3,000 milligrams of combined EPA plus DHA per day. This constitutes the daily maintenance dose I recommend as a preventive and for overall brain and body health. This usually means five capsules of good-quality fish oil (5,000 milligrams of fish oil liquid or capsules) per day. I know that sounds like a lot, but each 1,000 milligram capsule will contain smaller percentages of EPA plus DHA. This is what our bodies and brains need to reach

FISH OIL PRODUCT LABELS ARE CONFUSING! HERE'S A STEPWISE APPROACH TO READING A LABEL.

- Good products will tell you what the source of the fish oil is, like mackerel and sardines. They should be small feeder fish so there is less chance of bioaccumulation of toxins and heavy metals.
- Good products have on the label that it is molecularly distilled; that's the cleaning process to get rid of heavy metal and toxins.
- The suggested dose is usually one or two capsules. If it is two capsules, remember all amounts must be divided by two to determine the amount per capsule.
- Most capsules are 1,000 milligrams in size. They may tell you that there is 1,000 milligrams of fish oil or 1,000 milligrams of fat. If the serving size is two capsules, those amounts will be doubled, so 2,000 milligrams.
- Some capsules are 1,200 milligrams in size or 2,400 milligrams for two.
- Good products should provide a total of 500–600 milligrams of combined EPA+DHA per 1,000 milligram capsule.
- Great products will tell you that the omega-3s are in the triglyceride form. If the product isn't, they usually won't tell you, and you can expect that they are not. Manufacturing into triglyceride form is difficult and expensive, but the end product is worth the extra cost, with much less chance of side effects such as stomach upset.
- Recently, some new products are making it to the market that are in the good triglyceride form, 1,200 milligrams in size, but even more concentrated, and that provide 1,000 milligrams per capsule of combined EPA+DHA (or 2,000 milligrams in two capsules). Previously, the only concentrations that high were in a different, less tolerable form that often caused stomach upset or belching.

that healthy omega-3/omega-6 ratio. We need to reach that 3,000 milligram threshold and get to a 1:1 or 1:2 ratio.

A concussion raises the stakes, however. An injured brain suffering the waves of a biochemical cascade is going to need more anti-inflammatories and resolvins than an uninjured brain and quickly. Following a concussion, I highly recommend 3,000 milligrams of combined EPA+DHA three times per day. That's three doses of five capsules per day, or fifteen capsules, or 9,000 milligrams of combined EPA+DHA per day. This is essentially three times the normal, daily requirement. This nutritional support should start as soon as possible after the injury and continue for at least a week, or until symptoms abate, whichever is longer. After symptoms disappear, the patient should continue the protocol, decreasing to two doses of five capsules per day, or 6,000 milligrams of combined EPA+DHA daily, for another seven-day period. Even though symptoms may have disappeared at this point, there may still be some lingering inflammation, and this intermediary step is important. Finally, after a week longer on two doses of five capsules per day, the patient can resume or start with the daily dose of five capsules per day or 3,000 milligrams of combined EPA+DHA. I find people notice an improvement very quickly, often just a day or two after starting with such a high dose. This is encouraging, in and of itself, and makes patients more likely to continue to stay on the protocol.

THE OMEGA-3 PROTOCOL

STEP 1: Begin a high-quality omega-3 supplement—not all fish oil is the same (see resource section at the back of this book)

The omega-3 product should be a concentrated formulation that is molecularly distilled and pharmaceutical grade. The omega-3 product should be in triglyceride form preferably, not ethyl ester form, in order to decrease any unwanted digestion issues.

WHAT IS A DOSE? A single dose should be 3,000 milligrams of combined EPA+DHA. This works for most people age twelve and older.

For Capsules: Most high quality 1,000 milligrams soft gel capsules typically contain approximately 600 milligrams of EPA & DHA omega-3s combined.

In newer, more concentrated capsules like Nordic Naturals UltimateOmega 2X or ProOmega 2000, a dose would be three capsules, as each 1,250 milligram capsule provides 1,000 milligrams of combined EPA+DHA.

For Liquid: 1 to 1.5 teaspoons (5.0 to 7.5 ml) should contain approximately 3,000 milligrams of combined EPA+DHA.

For Re:Mind Recover: one 2-ounce bottle equals one dose.

WHAT ABOUT KIDS? To be more precise, a dose can be calculated as 40 milligrams of combined EPA+DHA per kilogram (18.2 milligrams of combined EPA+DHA per pound). This is helpful when dealing with children or anyone weighing less than one hundred pounds.

STEP 2: Begin taking your omega-3s as soon as possible following an injury as follows:

- Week 1: Take ONE dose THREE times a day for seven days (Breakfast-Lunch-Dinner or before work or school, after work or school, and at bedtime.
- Week 2: Take ONE dose TWO times a day for seven days.

IMPORTANT NOTE: If symptoms are improving, but not yet back to normal or where you and your health-care provider think you should be, strongly consider staying on these higher doses for a longer period of time until you achieve the results you believe you and your health-care provider believe you should achieve. Have a low threshold to go back up to a higher dose if symptoms return after going to a lower dose.

STEP 3: Continue with a maintenance dose to maintain optimal brain health. Continue to take approximately 3,000 milligrams of combined EPA+DHA every day.

This protocol has not been approved by the US Food and Drug Administration. The FDA has classified up to 3,000 milligrams of EPA+DHA omega-3 fatty acids as Generally Recognized as Safe (GRAS) without fear of adverse events. In addition, there are no known significant drug interactions with omega-3 fatty acids. When using higher amounts of EPA and DHA, it is important for persons considering doing this protocol to do so under the supervision of a health-care provider. Following this protocol does not constitute a doctor-patient relationship with Dr. Lewis, the clinical practice BrainCARE, or the Brain Health Education and Research Institute. It does not imply, explicitly or implicitly, any knowledge about your condition or that following the protocol is treating any medical condition for you.

I've challenged a number of "normal" people to try The Omega-3 Protocol just to experience its power. One person is the director of communications for the omega-3 industry organization. After a couple of days, she reported, "I am trying the TBI protocol and I have to say, I feel amazing. I started Wednesday morning so this is my third day and I can see why people don't go down to a lower dose. I normally take 2,200 milligrams of EPA and DHA, so this is a bit more than quadruple my regular dose. I feel great—mentally clear and with such a positive attitude—with no side effects. This is not a time of year I'm usually in a good mood—especially this winter—so it's great to feel such a mood benefit!"

It's not just healthy people, though. Concussion patients report clearer thinking, more energy, decreased headaches, less irritability, and a sense of calmness. Everyday life may have left them confused, headachy, forgetful, tired, and overwhelmed by the details of life. With The Omega-3 Protocol their condition will improve quickly, and they find they can return to normal activities and handle life and its challenges with a certain amount of grace. Take Josh, for example.

JOSH

Josh, a Marine, served during the initial invasion of Iraq in 2003. At one point, he was hit by an IED and knocked unconscious. He woke at the National Naval Medical

Center in Bethesda, Maryland, with a traumatic brain injury from the explosion. Eventually he recovered, and his enlistment was up. He was in the process of putting through his discharge paperwork to leave the service, when the US Marines called for a "stop loss" on all Marine infantrymen like Josh. A stop loss is the involuntary extension of a service member's active duty under the enlistment contract. The Marines were retaining Josh's services beyond the initial end of his term of service date. He was put on a plane and sent back to Iraq.

Five months later, while on a mission, he ran into trouble. On a raid, as he kicked in a door, his momentum carried him into the room. He saw an enemy combatant to his left. Before he could swing his weapon around, the man shot him at point-blank range. Because the shot was taken from the side, the bullet went under his body armor, entered his chest, and pierced his heart. Josh woke a second time in Bethesda. Somehow, the medic managed to keep him alive and Josh survived. This time when he recovered, Josh was medically retired from the Marines. He was free to leave service, find a job, and make a life for himself without the fear of being sent back into combat.

And he did find work. I met Josh when he sold me some windows. It was a hot day in August 2009, when my family moved into a new house. Well, it was technically not a new house, but a forty-year-old colonial with the original leaky windows. My wife and I wanted to have the windows replaced, and Josh was the salesperson. It took just a short time before the window brochures were pushed to the side and his story became the topic of conversation. He was medically retired, not just for getting shot in the heart, but for his traumatic brain injury that happened on the first deployment. I asked him if he still suffered with symptoms. Josh reported terrible headaches every single day, memory loss, and irritability.

"I'm the poster child for road rage on the Washington, DC, Beltway," he said by way of explaining his irritability and lack of patience. "And half the time when I go to appointments, I have to call back to the office because I don't remember where I'm going or where my next appointment is." He revealed that even outside of work, he often couldn't remember why he was in the car or what he should be doing while out on errands.

With our military brotherhood firmly established, I sat him down with two bottles: one of scotch, and one of fish oil. I said, "Take five fish oil capsules now. Wash them down with some scotch. Here's the bottle of fish oil. Take fifteen a day. Five in the morning, five at lunch, and five in the evening." He left, the Scotch glass empty and a full bottle of fish oil capsules tucked away in his pocket.

A few weeks later, the windows arrived and were installed. Soon after, Josh returned for a follow-up. On paper, his visit was to check the windows and make sure they were installed properly and that we were happy customers. For me, however, it was really an opportunity to gage his recovery. I wanted to hear if the fish oil had helped him and if he still suffered symptoms.

Josh reported zero headaches since the day he started taking fish oil. He quit calling into the office for directions and additional help because now he could remember his appointments. And when it came to the Beltway, he proclaimed: "I'm actually calm."

CONCUSSIONS ARE LIKE SNOWFLAKES

Omega-3s are not a miracle drug. Expectations must remain realistic when embarking on any treatment. What these fatty acids do is provide a nutritional foundation, what we call a neuropermissive environment so healing of the brain can occur.

Different recovery outcomes from concussion have to do with many variables. I like to say that concussions are like snowflakes. Everyone person, every injury, and every TBI is different—no two are alike. The extent of the injury is important, of course, but there are other variables as well. Who gleans the most benefit from fish oil and to what extent their brains can heal depends on age, gender, genetics, preexisting conditions, and how long ago the primary injury occurred. All these variables have an influence on why patients can heal at varying rates.

Age is certainly a determining factor. The very young and very old may have a harder time recovering from a brain injury than a healthy, twenty-five-year-old man. A child's brain is still forming. All the connections between different parts of the brain are still developing as well, and sections relegated to certain responsibilities—such as vision, hearing, memory, spatial awareness, and risk assessment—are all developing at different times. A child's or teen's neck muscles are also not as developed and leave the head more susceptible to brain injury. The head is large and heavy and needs a strong support. Without a strong neck, the head can be struck or can strike an object and a weak neck is left nearly useless to ameliorate the effects of the blow.

The brain also takes a while to mature. The last part of the brain to mature is the prefrontal cortex—the area of the brain that controls executive functioning, or how we control ourselves to make logical, good decisions. The male brain doesn't really finish this growth process until somewhere around twenty-five, believe it or not. Then, of course, as we get older, the brain becomes more fragile again. The neck weakens. The blood vessels become compromised and more susceptible to damage if an injury like a blow occurs.

Gender is another variable in concussion. Girls and women suffer concussion symptoms at a higher rate than boys and men. While a flood of attention has focused the spotlight on NFL players and helped create awareness of the health risks of concussion, girls' and women's sports are being overlooked. In many popular sports, boys are not the ones most likely afflicted by concussions—girls are. Across all sports played by both male and female athletes—such as soccer, ice hockey, basketball, lacrosse, and baseball/softball—female players experience concussions at a much higher rate than male players. In some cases, the rate is doubled, or more. While football gets all the attention in high school and college, the sport that has the highest rate of concussion in youth sports is female ice hockey.

A lot of attention has been directed toward the head and neck size of girls and the musculature of girls. Researchers speculate that girls have smaller, weaker necks than boys of the same age, and this leaves them more susceptible to trauma. Hormones could also play a role. If a teen or woman suffers a concussion in the premenstrual phase when progesterone levels are high, the injury will cause an abrupt drop in the hormone. That kind of immediate drop in progesterone can contribute to, or worsen, symptoms like headache, nausea, and dizziness, and trouble concentrating.

It has been estimated that the pituitary gland is affected in at least 30 percent of all head injuries, possibly as high as 70 to 80 percent. The pituitary gland controls hormones and their influence on the body, including growth hormone, the thyroid, and the sex hormones: progesterone, estrogen, and testosterone. It's not uncommon to see problems with any or all of these hormones in both males and females after concussion.

Preexisting conditions, whether physical or mental, also can affect the outcomes of concussion. If coupled with a head injury, those suffering with ADHD, depression, autism, anxiety disorders, and other mental illnesses often have a much more difficult time recovering. Brain function is already compromised in these individuals, and concussion exacerbates an already stressed system. It's sad, but I've seen instances where medical insurance companies will refuse to cover a person's TBI because of these "pre-existing conditions," when they should recognize that they make TBI much more difficult to recover and need more medical assistance, not less.

Genetically, some people may be more susceptible to injury than others. For example, there is some evidence to suggest that the gene that's linked to risk of Alzheimer's is also an indicator of higher risk of having difficulty recovering from head injuries or having more severe symptoms if and when an injury occurs. People with this gene also are thought less capable of a full recovery after a head injury.

The length of time between the primary injury and beginning The Omega-3 Protocol is certainly a variable. Obviously, you want to begin The Omega Protocol as soon as possible after the primary injury, but that should not dissuade patients from supplementing their diets with fish oil months or even years after their accident (or before). Maintaining that balance, that healthy ratio between omega-3s and omega-6s, should be a lifelong commitment. In terms of brain trauma with persisting symptoms over time, I often hear the question, "My injury was years ago—do you think The Omega Protocol might still help me?"

What I have found is, yes, it can help. The more severe or the longer ago the injury, the longer a person may need to be on the higher dose of omega-3s to help the brain recover. Remember, omega-3s are nutrition. You don't stop eating a certain food group because you feel better. This is nutrition for life. In severely injured patients or patients who suffer from lasting effects of concussion over years, any benefits gained will be lost if omega-3s are withheld or reduced. At this point, supporting the brain nutritionally is what will allow the brain to heal and function optimally.

MARIO

Mario was a fit, strong twenty-five-year-old who went out rock climbing on New Year's Eve in 2011 at Joshua Tree National Monument. He is described by his mother as the kind of guy who is always "very healthy and athletic. He's a bicycle enthusiast. He's ridden his bike across the country from California to Virginia. Alone." Mario was clearly in peak physical condition at the time of his fall.

When climbing, somehow his feet got tangled up in

gear, and he lost his grip and fell, hitting his head. He lay in a coma for a week before regaining consciousness and was then transferred to a rehabilitation hospital. After months of convalescing, he was finally discharged, allowed to come home, and told his brain had healed.

For the next ten months, Mario suffered with constant, debilitating headaches, memory problems, challenges with executive functioning, and damage to the optic nerve, which affected his vision. His mother reached out to me through my nonprofit website, described Mario's fall, and explained, "My son didn't just have a concussion. He suffered a severe TBI. He almost died. He broke his skull in seventeen places, had emergency brain surgery to remove a blood clot, was in a coma for more than a week, and trauma ICU for more than a month, before we could move him."

I forwarded The Omega Protocol and followed up with his mom. Mario took high-dose fish oil for one and a half months. Then one day, I got an email direct from Mario himself. When Mario had started the protocol, he explained, "I'd been having headaches nearly every day and hydrocodone did nothing for me. Headaches come out of nowhere and don't go away for at least a week. Since I started taking fish oil, my headaches are gone."

Mario discovered that if he missed a dose, or tried a lower dosage, "I can truly feel the mental differences." For him, it meant that his short-term memory was not as good if he didn't take his fish oil. Mario continued reporting to me directly as his recovery continued. Two months later, I received an email where he confessed, "If I don't have omega-3, I'm DEAD! It has turned my life completely around."

The last I heard from Mario, he was doing great. He wanted me to come out and talk to the Brain Injury Association of California (BIACAL) and explain how The Omega Protocol works, why it works, and how to feed the brain what it needs. All common sense. Right?

CHAPTER SIX

THE USE OF OMEGA-3S IN SEVERE BRAIN INJURY

GAIL

Gail and Philip were in their sixties. They both worked for the government, Philip as a lawyer, and Gail as the Deputy Director of Early Childhood Education for the Department of Education. Philip retired before Gail, at the end of August 2012. On the first day of his retirement, September 1, the couple was traveling up through Pennsylvania en route to their weekend house for a mini vacation. They came around the corner on the interstate and there was a police car stopped right in the middle of the highway. Philip swerved to avoid hitting the police officer, went off the road, lost control, and the car overturned.

Gail was asleep in the backseat. Philip, wearing his seatbelt, escaped unharmed, but Gail was severely injured and was air evacuated to the nearest trauma center. She was not expected to live. By mid-October, she was still in a coma, but had stabilized enough to transfer her to a rehabilitation facility in Baltimore to be closer to home. Her daughter, Suzanne, who was also a lawyer in Baltimore, had just watched CNN's Sanjay Gupta special about Bobby, the young teenager in the terrible car accident described at the beginning of the book. Bobby's accident and recovery was the subject of an in-depth story where Julian Bailes and I were featured, linking the Sago Mine disaster and Bobby's journey, and explaining how fish oil was crucial to the recovery of both Randy McCloy and Bobby. The show aired on October 20, nearly two months after Gail's accident.

The following week, Suzanne reached out to me. Gail's doctors agreed to try the protocol, but they needed to know where and what kind of fish oil to purchase and how much to give her. I provided answers and forwarded the protocol for severe TBI using high-dose fish oil. They started that day.

Gail was sixty-one years old. Her discharge summary from the trauma hospital listed twenty-nine separate diagnoses including diffuse subarachnoid hemorrhage, diffuse axonal injury, severe injuries to multiple parts of the brain, and bone fractures of everything from her ribs to spine. Even on her arrival to the rehabilitation facility, the consulting neurologist told the family: "Unfortunately I am not optimistic that we will see substantial amount of additional improvement" in Gail. The doctors told Philip there was less than a 10 percent chance Gail would ever regain consciousness. This was the baseline from which we started.

Once Gail received omega-3s, she immediately improved. Her daughter reported that her mother regained consciousness around Christmas and was learning how to walk, how to swallow, and she could sit up. In February, I received an email from Suzanne detailing how her mother's recovery far exceeded anyone's expectations. She was fully conscious at this point, talking and even making jokes. She's nowhere near 100 percent, but she continues to makes strides in her recovery.

Gail's recovery timeline was impressive given the extent and seriousness of her injuries. September 1 was the day of the terrible accident. In late October, I was contacted and Gail began to receive omega-3s, two months after the accident. Then three months later, five months in all since that nightmarish day, Gail was conscious and progressing with acquiring speech and walking. Even the well-respected neurologist in Baltimore, who assessed

Gail back in November and carefully explained to Philip and Suzanne how Gail would never improve beyond a persistent vegetative state, could not believe how well she recovered. The neurologist now believes omega-3s most certainly played a factor.

SEVERE TRAUMA TBI AND DIFFUSE AXONAL INJURY

Severe traumatic brain injury (TBI) is a major cause of death and disability in the United States, contributing to about 30 percent of all injury deaths. Every day, 138 people in the United States die from injuries that include TBI. Those who survive a TBI can face effects lasting a few days to disabilities that often persist the rest of their lives. Effects of TBI can include impaired thinking or memory, movement, sensation (vision or hearing), or emotional functioning (personality changes, depression, and/or anxiety disorders), among others. These issues not only affect individuals but can have lasting impacts on families and communities, and the economic consequences can be devastating.

A TBI is caused by a bump, blow, or jolt to the head, or a penetrating head injury that disrupts the normal function of the brain. Not all blows or jolts to the head result in a TBI, though. The severity of a TBI may range from "mild" (i.e., a brief change in mental status or consciousness) to "severe" (i.e., an extended period of unconsciousness or memory loss after the injury). Most TBIs that occur each

TBI IN THE UNITED STATES

Estimated Average Annual Number of Traumatic Brain Injury-Related Emergency Department Visits, Hospitalizations, and Deaths: 2002–2006

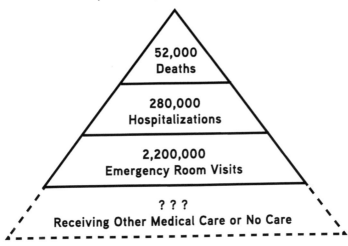

52,000
Deaths

280,000
Hospitalizations

2,200,000
Emergency Room Visits

? ? ?
Receiving Other Medical Care or No Care

SOURCE cdc.gov

year are mild, and these are what we call concussions. A severe TBI is often what results in coma, severe brain inflammation, disability, and sometimes death.

When TBI is more severe, symptoms last longer, and many times there is permanent impairment. The extent of these kinds of injuries is profound, and the number of victims is staggering. A quick look at the numbers is sobering:

- TBI contributed to the deaths of more than 50,000 people annually.
- Each year, TBI is a diagnosis in more than 280,000 hospitalizations and 2.2 million emergency visits. These consisted of

TBI alone or TBI in combination with other injuries.

- Over the past decade (2001–2010), while rates of TBI-related emergency visits increased by 70 percent, hospitalization rates only increased by 11 percent and death rates decreased by 7 percent.
- From 2001 to 2009, the rate of emergency department visits for sports and recreation-related injuries with a diagnosis of concussion or TBI, alone or in combination with other injuries, rose 57 percent among children (age nineteen or younger).

LEADING CAUSES OF TBI

The most recent compilation of statistics come from 2006–2010. In that period, falls were the leading cause of TBI, accounting for 40 percent of all TBIs in the United States that resulted in an emergency visit, hospitalization, or death. Falls disproportionately affect the youngest and oldest age groups, which makes sense as these are always our most vulnerable populations. More than half (55%) of TBIs among children from birth to fourteen years old are caused by falls. More than two-thirds (81%) of TBIs in adults aged sixty-five and older are caused by falls. What we call "unintentional blunt trauma," like being struck in the head by a baseball bat or a helmet, is the second leading cause of TBI (15%). When we break it down further, close to a quarter of all TBIs in children less than fifteen years old are the result of blunt trauma.

LEADING CAUSES OF TBI

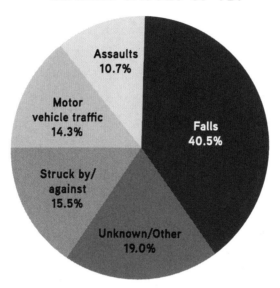

SOURCE http://www.cdc.gov/traumaticbraininjury/get_the_facts.html

Among all age groups, motor vehicle crashes are the third overall leading cause of TBI (14%).

Mortality rates can also be assessed. When looking at just TBI-related deaths, motor vehicle crashes are the second leading cause of TBI-related deaths at 26 percent. Roughly 10 percent of all lethal TBIs are due to assaults. They accounted for 3 percent of TBIs in children under fifteen and 1.4 percent of TBIs in adults sixty-five and older. About 75 percent of all lethal assaults associated with TBI occur in people fifteen to forty-four.

In general, men are nearly three times as likely to die

as women from severe TBI, and rates were highest for the elderly sixty-five and older, with falls leading as the cause of the accident. Motor vehicle crashes are the leading cause of death for children and young adults, five to twenty-four, and, tragically, assaults were the leading cause for children from birth to four years old.

Among nonfatal TBI-related injuries, men routinely have higher rates of TBI hospitalizations and emergency visits than women. Hospitalization rates were highest among the elderly years and very young children, again from birth to four years old.

These statistics are not meant to frighten parents or families. Rather, my intention is to demonstrate how widespread these accidents are and how common concussion and severe TBI are in our country. Let's hope you and your loved ones never have to deal with this kind of injury. But being prepared is important.

CONSIDERING THE OMEGA PROTOCOL FOR SEVERE TBI

As with any traumatic brain injury, The Omega Protocol should be considered as soon as possible after the initial accident. One of the worst issues with a severe TBI is what we call diffuse axonal injury (DAI). Remember, the brain is not just a homogenous bowl of jelly but is comprised of complicated structures within structures within structures, all of varying densities. A sudden, abrupt movement, a blow, or deceleration that makes the head stop creates the trauma. Here, the brain keeps moving, creating a shearing effect as the different structures of the brain tear away from each other based on their densities, and twisting and stretching neurons as the brain slams against the inside of the skull.

What can happen is those connections between the different parts of the brain, those axons, are damaged. Picture a neuron, a bundle of tissue with a star-like quality to it. Typically, there is one long arm off of the central body that reaches out like a tree branch to touch other neurons. That long branch is called an axon. Those axons are the connections between the different neurons or brain cells. In an accident, where the structures of the brain are moving at different speeds, those axons between the different parts of the brain are stretched. When they stretch too much, they can get twisted, or they can be literally sheared off completely. When this shearing is pervasive, across the entire brain, we call this DAI.

This is exactly the kind of serious injury a CT scan in the emergency room will fail to identify. Often, a week after an accident, an MRI will reveal DAI as white or bright spots around the brain where there is shearing. The person will most likely be in a coma or in an induced coma. That secondary biochemical cascade is at work, clearing dead tissue. The axons are stretched and some may die right away, but the largest percentage will die off later. It is the secondary injury, the biochemical cascade, that can

CT SCAN AT TIME OF INJURY:
NO DAI PRESENT

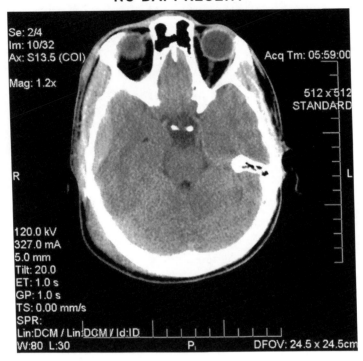

MRI ONE WEEK LATER:
DAI PRESENT

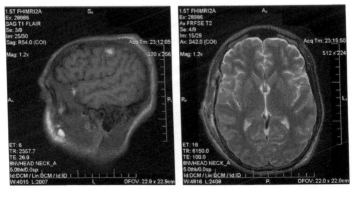

cause further cell death, which can lead to complications. That inflammatory effect, as necessary as it is to help the brain, if left unchecked, can even lead to further damage or even death.

CONVINCING YOUR DOCTOR

You may have to have a tantrum. If you are in the turmoil of an emergency involving a loved one, and especially if it's your child, you are going to feel marginalized by fear, the enormity of the situation, and the expertise of highly trained health-care professionals including neurologists, surgeons, doctors, and nursing staff. And the overwhelming, almost paralyzing feeling, is one of grief.

In my experience, what typically happens is the doctors will tell the family there is nothing more they can do and that only time will heal the brain. Quite often, if the injury is severe enough, the doctors will say, "There's no meaningful chance of recovery. Have you discussed organ donation?" As a parent, you can appreciate the horror of being told to pull the plug and end your child's life, but these are the words often used.

I've heard them. In the past, I've said them. This is one reason why I would love to be able to change how medicine is practiced. Doctors should think about providing a neuropermissive environment with optimal nutrition to give their patient's brain the best opportunity to heal, but that's not how they are trained. Sometimes it may help.

Sometimes it may not.

The visceral reaction from parents is almost universal: "I'll do anything to help my child." Nowadays you bring your laptop to the hospital, join their Wi-Fi, get onto the Internet, and start asking everybody everything: *What can be done for traumatic brain injury?* That's how people find me: literally, through search engines. That's why I get one thousand hits a day on my website.

Parents and family members learn about omega-3s. They ask their doctor. Unfortunately, more often than not, doctors put up resistance. They say nutritional treatments are experimental, or there's no scientific evidence that omega-3s work, and administering such high does could pose serious health risks. The reality is, they don't know enough about omega-3s. Their own lack of knowledge in this regard becomes the cement they use to create roadblocks. Rather than do something different, they will choose to do nothing. The doctors would rather choose to do nothing, than to move forward with a treatment that puts them out of their comfort zone.

If your son or daughter or loved one is suffering from severe brain trauma and DAI, I will tell you exactly what I tell families seeking my help: "The doctors, the nurses, the hospital staff, all go home at the end of their shift. You are there 24/7 because your loved one is lying there. You are investing far more time in your loved one's care than the hospital staff. You, as the family member, have to be more adamant about administering fish oil than your doctors are about putting roadblocks up." In some cases, family members have had to go to hospital administration or hire lawyers to force the hospitals to allow nutritional support with fish oil. What is most amazing to me is that we are talking about nutrition, not some crazy experimental drug!

I believe in practice and being prepared. In order to prepare for the worst, I will offer a template for action if you ever find yourself in a position where you are advocating for a loved one and trying to convince your doctor, your surgeon, and perhaps administrators, this is only nutrition. Omega-3s are not some experimental drug.

Scenario: You get a call from the hospital that your son or daughter been in an accident. By the time you arrive, your child may have already been moved for emergency surgery. Basically, the first time you will see your child might be in the intensive care unit, the ICU. Doctors may be around, but the nurses are omnipresent.

You find the ICU. The doctors will pull you aside or sit you down in a small conference room with no magazines. Though they sound caring, they will spell out the situation in clear, precise language with scary numbers. Your child has been in a very severe car accident. There's very little, less than 10 percent, chance of any meaningful recovery. Your child will probably never regain consciousness. You should probably consider allowing some good to come of this and think now about permitting organ donation. We have paperwork you can read.

It's 3:00 in the morning. You thought your teenager was out at a high school dance. Now he or she seems almost unrecognizable under a pile of tubes connected to machines. Under stress, you will feel marginalized by fear and grief. But there is also that visceral call to do something. Use it. And when the doctor repeats how there's really nothing further that can be done, how there's little hope of any kind of meaningful recovery, you ask about administering fish oil.

One of three things will happen. The doctors will agree. They'll look into it. They'll refuse. If they agree, be ready with the protocol and supply the fish oil. Most, if not all hospitals, will not have good-quality liquid fish oil in their pharmacy. If they plan to investigate further, send them to brainhealtheducation.org, which is listed in the resource section. If they refuse or say something as reported by one patient: "No, I'm not to do that; it's not safe. I'm familiar with this protocol. It could cause a lot of damage," ask to see their supervisor. You keep moving up the chain of command until you get what you want and what your child needs. You have to be more aggressive to force treatment than hospital administrators are to remain passive and do nothing.

Here's a script that can guide you:

"There's no way to know if omega-3s will help, but what

research shows is that the brain needs to be saturated with high doses of omega-3s in order to heal. Without an optimal supply of omegas, healing is less likely to happen. Omega-3s are not a drug and not a cure. Omegas may have a positive impact on neuroprotection of brain cells, neuroinflammation, and neuroregeneration. The brain needs a neuropermissive environment to be able to heal. I understand that every situation is different and some people may respond better than others. However, there's absolutely no downside to providing optimal levels of nutrition in order to give my child the best opportunity to regain as much function as possible."

Then offer this book or the links to stories mentioned in this book, the Sago Mine disaster, Bobby's story with Sanjay Gupta, and scientific articles and bibliographies published on BHERI's website. Explain the dose and duration. For severe brain trauma, the doses are much higher than the recommended dose found on any bottle. Those patients need 1 tablespoon or 15 milliliters twice a day for a total of 30 milliliters per day through the feeding tube, followed by a saline or salt-water flush. This dose was based on the amounts used on the survivor of the Sago Mine accident and Bobby's experience. Other patients have received this dose for more than a year without any health risks or side effects.

If the doctors do not initially agree, it may be hard. You may not feel like the expert, but in this case, you are your loved one's most ardent supporter. If there is a time to fight for your child or loved one, it is now. The good news is that with so much recent press and research, the kind of resistance involving legal recourse is slowly disappearing. More doctors and neurologists are learning about the effects and positive outcomes of omega-3s on the brain and in healing brain trauma. But to become mainstream, it is going to take more time, more experience, and more parents pushing doctors to try. In my experience, if a patient is going to come out of a coma, he or she will become responsive typically between two weeks and two months. When that happens, you will have better prepared your loved one for optimal brain healing.

Be firm.

Be persistent.

Be prepared.

LIQUID FISH OIL VIA FEEDING TUBE OR IV

Over the past couple of years, I have over one thousand people who have contacted me through my nonprofit. I don't know the exact number, just the exact number of emails, and as of today's writing, that's about 950. Once somebody starts asking questions and I respond, I'm not good about shutting down communication. I want to hear about the outcomes, improvements, how quickly they recovered. I want to hear their stories and the stories of their families so that I may share their experience with others going through a similar situation, or connect them with a support network of people. Brain trauma affects everyone in the family and, often, the community. Most people ask about how much fish oil to take or to give to their loved one, or if their concussion was twenty years ago, whether fish oil will help with seemingly chronic symptoms, like headaches and brain fog. Many of the questions have to do with how to give the fish oil, and the mechanics of administering the oil itself, especially to patients in a coma.

If a person is in a coma suffering from DAI, he or she should receive 15 milliliters twice a day or 30 milliliters a day. A good-quality liquid fish oil concentrate should provide almost 10,000 milligrams of EPA and almost 8,000 milligrams of DHA for a total of around 19,000 to 20,000 milligrams of omega-3s daily. The bottle typically will tell you the dosage is 1 teaspoon (5 ml) a day, providing around 3,000 milligrams of combined EPA and DHA. Because you will triple that, the way to administer this is through a feeding tube, and then have the nurses clear the line with a saline flush. Unfortunately, there is currently no way to administer fish oil through an IV. Fish oil is, in fact, oil—and oil and water don't mix, right? If you were to put oil into an IV, the patient would not survive simply because oil clumps and blood vessels would be blocked, compromised, and destroyed.

While these doses were used in adults, in pediatric

patients, lower doses should be considered. A very rudimentary, completely untested and arbitrary rule would be to divide the patient's weight by ten to give the total number of milliliters of UltimateOmega twice per day. For example, in a 100 lb child, 10 milliliters should be considered twice a day for a total of 20 milliliters per day. For a more precise calculation, that would be 120 milligrams of combined EPA+DHA per kilogram to be given twice per day (or 55 milligrams of combined EPA+DHA per pound to be given twice per day).

These protocols should only be used under the guidance of an attending physician and monitored with a fatty-acid profile analysis on a weekly basis.

Ironically, the only two intravenous nutrition products approved in the United States are both soybean oil based. Now that you are the expert, you know this means these products have essentially no omega-3s but a large amount of pro-inflammatory omega-6s. Again, that would worsen the imbalance favoring the inflammatories, putting the body and the brain on track for escalating secondary injuries.

Mark Puder, MD, PhD, a pediatric surgeon at Boston Children's Hospital, treats premature infants suffering from short bowel syndrome (SBS) or short gut syndrome. SBS is a malabsorption disorder with myriad causes from the surgical removal of the small intestine to congenital deformities. In some premature babies, the gut has not

SEVERE TBI PROTOCOL

- Adults with a severe TBI in a coma and/or reliant on a feeding tube
  - → 15 milliliters twice a day of high quality, concentrated omega-3 fish oil (30 milliliters total per day)
  - → That amount of a good-quality liquid fish oil concentrate should provide about 10,000 milligrams of EPA and 8,000 milligrams of DHA for a total of 18,000 to 22,000 milligrams of omega-3s daily

- Children or pediatric doses
  - → Divide the child's weight by 10 to give the total number of milliliters of high quality, concentrated omega-3 fish oil twice per day. For example, in a 50 lb child, 5 milliliters should be considered twice a day for a total of 10 milliliters per day.
  - → For a more precise calculation, 120 milligrams of combined EPA+DHA per kilogram to be given twice per day (240 mg/kg total daily) or 55 milligrams of combined EPA+DHA per pound to be given twice per day (10 mg/lb total daily)

- These protocols should only be used under the guidance of an attending physician and monitored with a fatty-acid profile analysis on a weekly basis until levels are stable
  - → The overall omega-6:omega-3 ratio should be brought down under 5:1 but not below 1:1
  - → The AA:EPA ratio should be brought down to around 1.5

- Bleeding is not a concern at these levels and can be used safely with "blood thinning" pharmaceuticals such as heparin completely formed and is left unable to absorb nutrients. In this case, even a feeding tube is useless as the infant still cannot absorb nutrients offered. Basically, physicians are left with the choice of feeding the infant through an IV or not at all. This means the infant will receive nutritional supplements intravenously loaded with soybean oil and omega-6s.

This imbalance creates a fatty liver, or what is called Parenteral Nutrition-Associated Liver Disease (PNALD), and the child will die from liver disease if left on the formula too long. What Dr. Puder has discovered is that fish-oil based IV lipid emulsions can prevent and/or reverse the effects of PNALD. Dr. Puder continues to study PNALD and is only allowed by the FDA to use the fish-oil based emulsions on an experimental basis. He has to import one of three different emulsions from Europe, where these are approved. These emulsions contain fish oil in significant quantities in the IV nutrition.

Short gut syndrome is essentially 100 percent fatal if the child receives no intervention. The problem is that the current intervention is nearly as dangerous. With currently approved IV nutrition products based on soybean oil, it becomes a race. Is the IV nutrition going to kill the child, or will the infant's gut mature quickly enough that it can be fed by regular formula? Using the fish-oil based products, however, has been more successful than Dr. Puder predicted. Dr. Puder's results using fish oil with these little babies has been so positive that the scientific community and other pediatricians find the figures difficult to believe. As Dr. Puder once told me, "The results are so unbelievable, no one believes it."

If there are three fish-oil-based nutritional products already produced and approved in Europe, I questioned, how do we maximize the amount of omega-3s in one of those IV products so we can use it here in the United States for TBI? This was one of the first questions that came into my mind when I first thought about using omega-3s for head-injured military patients. In terms of military applications, the question I had was: How many omega-3s can fit in a 20 milliliter syringe a medic could carry in his medical kit on the battlefield in Iraq or Afghanistan? As soon as IV access is established, omega-3s could be administered and help jump-start the process of brain healing right there at the scene of the injury. Then, once you get the injured soldier to the combat hospital, you can start an intravenous drip to continue to provide that vital nutrition to the soldier's brain. In the civilian world, this would mean the EMT would have it available in the back of an ambulance for immediate use, and in the emergency room you could start the IV drip. Developing this protocol for the Army is one of the current projects I am still involved with in terms of military, frontline medicine.

As of today's writing, there is no way to offer patients omega-3s via IV. I thought when I came up with this idea and started the process, we'd have the product through the onerous FDA process by now. I couldn't be more wrong. The IV product I invented is still stuck going through animal testing. With further research and investment, hopefully this will change. At this point, the only way to administer omega-3s is through a feeding tube followed by a saline flush.

In closing, remember, omega-3s are not the silver magic bullet that's going to reverse brain injury. These fatty acids provide the optimal nutritional foundation to balance the inflammatory response, start the resolution process following inflammation, and allow the brain to heal if, and this is a big *if*, the brain is going to heal. Omega-3s may have a positive impact on neuroprotection of brain cells, neuroinflammation, and neuroregeneration. Every situation is different, and some people may respond better than others. For some the damage may be too extensive. However, there is no downside to providing optimal levels of nutrition in order to give the patient the best opportunity to regain as much function as possible. Keep expectations realistic.

THE MEDICAL COMMUNITY

The American Society for Parenteral and Enteral Nutrition (ASPEN) ("parenteral" means intravenous nutrition and "enteral" means nutrition with a feeding tube), the European Society for Parenteral and Enteral Nutrition (ESPEN), and the Society for Critical Care Medicine (SCCM) offer guidelines for critically ill adults.

These guidelines change every year or two. The 2015 guidelines for nutritional-support therapy in adult critically ill patients cover both parenteral and enteral treatment. Of those guidelines, there were only two recommendations that rated highest according to the quality of evidence. This meant there were only two recommendations out of thirty-four that had received what's called a grade A recommendation based on supported evidence. The only two recommendations getting a grade A recommendation both pertained to offering patients nutrition that includes omega-3s. "Based on expert consensus we suggest the use of immune modulating formulations or EPA/DHA supplement with standard enteral formula and patients with traumatic brain injury."

For the first time, in February 2016, the ASPEN and SCCM published a separate set of nutritional recommendations for traumatic brain injury and concussion. Previously, there were no specific recommendations specifically for TBI. Now, both agencies and their cousin in Europe, ESPEN, specifically state that the use of EPA and DHA in neurologically injured populations has recently gained significant attention and accelerates recovery after traumatic brain injury. The guidelines lay it out: "Based on expert consensus, we suggest the use of either arginine containing immune modulating formulations or EPA/DHA supplement with standard enteral formula and patients with TBI."

Though this is encouraging, the reality is these guidelines are not followed by medical practitioners. Doctors usually don't know about them or read the updated material and tend to follow what they were taught in school and residency training. It's an education process for doctors. Think of how children are educated. If you look at what kids are learning in New York, the curriculum may be a little bit different than what they're learning in Mississippi versus what they're learning in rural New Mexico on an Indian reservation. It's still high school, it's still tenth grade, but what they're learning can be different. It's not a whole lot different in concept from how doctors are educated. There are regional differences and differences between medical schools and residency training programs.

If your child or loved one is injured and suffering from concussion or a severe TBI, you may have to step in and model the role of an educator. This may not be comfortable, and reactions will vary. You may not feel welcome at the table—or, hopefully, you might be surprised at the level of cooperation. The range of acceptance for nutritional treatment is wide and each medical case presents its own challenges from the injury itself to how care is managed.

There are times when I find myself questioning if I'm making a difference. After all, I couldn't get the US Army to listen to me when I did a published study with the NIH on how omega-3s might reduce suicides in our soldiers. Julian Bailes and I published a paper in *Military Medicine* advocating for use of fish oil to increase the resilience of the brain to withstand injury in the first place. Then I had published the story of Bobby in a medical journal and it was picked up as a great story by Sanjay Gupta. There are times when it seems like all I get are emails from people asking, "How do I get the doctors to try omega-3s in my child who is in a coma?" It can be frustrating for the families but also for me. I don't have all the answers. Ask the doctors to follow the ASPEN critical-care guidelines.

Just when I'm reaching a level of frustration and wondering if I am making a difference, I get an email that renews my faith that what I'm doing is helping, even if it is just one TBI patient at a time. I want to share a few emails with you that I've received over the past few years. I hope that you will never be in this situation, but if you are facing the possibility of a loved one struggling to survive a severe TBI, I pray these emails, in their own unedited words, will give you hope:

I emailed you back in October regarding my sixty-one-year-old mother who sustained severe diffuse axonal brain injury from an accident. She, like Bobby Ghassemi, was at a Glasgow coma score of 3 in the hospital and was not expected to survive (she also sustained 15 broken bones). After she did survive, the doctors told my father that she would never improve and there was a less than 10% chance of regaining consciousness. We started her on your recommended does of omega-3 on October 27, 2012.

I'm happy to say that she's far exceeded anyone's expectations. She is currently fully conscious (full of life), alert, and talking (she's even cracking jokes). She regained full consciousness right around Christmas. She's in subacute rehabilitation. She's relearning to walk, swallow, and other basic life skills. She exceeded everyone's expectations, even a well-respected neurologist in the area who assessed her back in November and told us that she wouldn't improve much beyond her persistent vegetative state. The doctor on her floor believes that the "omega-3 certainly played a factor."

Here is another:

My son was a pedestrian hit by a car at pretty high speed on September 20, 2012. He had a Glasgow scale of 3. He was not expected to survive. When he did survive, the doctors were sure he would remain in a vegetative state. I saw the article on CNN about fish oil and asked his doctor to consider it. He reviewed the article and agreed to try it.

My son had a Diffuse Axonal Injury and a frontal lobe brain injury. He made a remarkable recovery! We used the amounts mentioned in the article. Everyone should use this for a brain injury.

And another:

My son was in a horrific car accident on August 3, 2013. The doctors at the hospital gave him little hope as his brain had suffered terrible trauma. They called it brain shearing. They think he rolled somewhere between 4 and 6 times. Everything they did was negative; MRIs, CTs, and the EEG showed basically nothing. I decided I couldn't just sit by his bed and cry and started searching the internet for recovery stories, and I found the two about the fish oil and you. By now after almost 3 weeks in ICU and now in a next level down I talked to the family about the fish oil and everyone agreed let's talk to the doctors. The nurse advocated for us and they started giving it to him a week ago on August 25. On Thursday, August 29, his wife asked him if he was in pain just talking to him and he shook his head no. We both almost fell over. We always felt he heard us but the doctors kept saying it was nothing when we thought he squeezed our hand or seemed agitated. They said if he ever woke up he wouldn't recognize or remember anything. On Friday, August 29, they took his trach out that morning because he was breathing fine on his own. Early that afternoon surrounded by his wife, me, and some other family members he started trying to talk. Very scared and frustrated because he can't see and he kept mumbling get me outta here. Well it's

Sunday, September 1, and my son is laying in his hospital bed resting in front of me. His wife stayed the night in his room last night and this morning although his jaw is very sore as it was broke in the accident he could tell the nurse's name from yesterday and the month and year. We are overjoyed. I want to make sure my son has every possible option for recovery. He is 25 years old and had just gotten married on July 20, 2013, and had 2 beautiful kids. Thank goodness for God and prayers and leading me to the Bobby Ghassami story and you. Look forward to hearing from you. We are very early in his recovery and want to make sure we do everything we can for him. It was only 4 weeks ago last night that I got the call that every parent is scared of. Thank you again.

And a final note:

Hi Dr. Lewis,

I believe my mother reached out to you in the past regarding your work with Omega-3 Fish Oil and the positive impact it has on people who have had brain injuries. I unfortunately had a severe accident on Halloween, and fell a significant distance which caused me to suffer a Traumatic Brain Injury. I was forced to have surgery on my head to reduce the ICP on my brain, and was in a coma for a couple of weeks. In the time I spent at the hospital I made a significant recovery and left the hospital on March 2. Part of this recovery was obviously the therapy I was doing in the hospital, but I believe that it was my consumption of Omega-3s that drove my relatively fast recovery.

I just wanted to thank you for all of the important work that you all have put into researching Omega-3s and the impact that it has on the brain. I believe that the impact it made on my recovery has caused some doctors here in Calgary to believe that Omega-3 consumption should be included for the treatment of others with brain injuries.

Thank you again for all your hard work as it made a significant difference on my life.

CHAPTER SEVEN

IT'S NEVER TOO EARLY: OMEGA-3S AS PREVENTIVE MEDICINE

Virtually everyone should be taking a maintenance dose of fish oil for a variety of reasons. But to help prevent concussion and better prepare the brain in case of injury, two populations stand out as more at risk of concussion and in need of pre-injury care: soldiers and athletes.

In 2011, Dr. Julian Bailes and I coauthored and published a journal article in *Military Medicine*. "Neuroprotection for the Warrior: Dietary Supplementation with Omega-3 Fatty Acids" advocated that soldiers and athletes, really anyone who is at risk of a head injury, should be taking 3,000 milligrams of the EPA+DHA, or the daily dose the FDA recognizes as safe. This maintenance dose improves the resilience of the brain to withstand injury. If an injury were to occur, the brain would already be balanced with the right ratio of omega-3s to omega-6s to help dampen secondary injuries and begin the healing process immediately. A powerful example of the preventive power of omega-3s is Elijah Sedig's story. In his own words, following are the emails this young man sent me while deployed to Afghanistan.

ELIJAH'S THIRD COMBAT DEPLOYMENT AS AN EOD BOMB TECH

7/3/12

I'm currently deployed to Afghanistan as an EOD technician and my mom saw your program and buys fish oil and sends it to me. I have been taking the fish oil since I got the first package from her about two weeks into my deployment. I have been about 50 meters from 320 pounds of explosives when it detonated and I watched a grenade detonate no more than ten feet in front of me. I have never experienced any sort of postconcussive symptoms when everyone around me at those times has had some sort of headache or other TBI-type symptoms... One of the medical personnel at the Kandahar Airfield Hospital said that it's good genetics but I'm not convinced (even though I do have impeccable blood lines hahahaha)... If there is other information I might be able to help with, let me know and I would be more than happy to.

Respectfully,
SSG Elijah Sedig
EOD Team Leader
741st Ordnance Company (EOD)

7/12/12
I gave a bottle of the GNC DHA 600 pills to another team leader who has been entirely too close to at least three detonations (IEDs went off while he was interrogating them with a grappling hook from something like ten feet), so I will let you know how they work for him!

8/12/12
I'm doing well, tired of being deployed and more than ready to be home but still taking fish oil. I haven't had any sort of indication that it is anything other than awesome. I think I told you before that I know I have depression I just have never been diagnosed with it and I noticed that I haven't been depressed this entire deployment so I believe that is because of the fish oil. Thanks for checking in!!

3/23/13
I'm sorry that I have taken my sweet time in getting back to you! I have meant to respond to you for quite some time and I will make the time now!

While I was preparing for my deployment my mother (a dietician at the VA hospital in Tucson, Arizona) read an article about a study that showed that omega-3 fatty acids could possibly help people recover from concussions or traumatic brain injury (TBI). Because I was preparing for a deployment to Afghanistan as an Explosive Ordnance Disposal (EOD) Team Leader and I was absolutely going to be near many improvised explosive devices (IEDs), she told me that she was going to send me omega-3s and the DVD from Dr. Lewis. It took her a little bit longer than she meant for it to come, so for about the first month I wasn't taking any omega-3 supplements. During that time, I was on an operation where several people were approximately twenty to thirty feet from a forty-pound cratering charge when it detonated, knocking them unconscious. After I received my first box from my mother with several bottles of GNC DHA 600, I heard one of the guys talking about how he was having severe headaches and other symptoms of serious TBI. I told him about the article my mother had read and I gave him a bottle of the pills. I saw him the next day as we were walking around camp and he told me that he had woken up with a much less severe headache, and for the first time in weeks he was actually able to get out of bed almost immediately without being disoriented or blinded by the headache. This was my first real experience with someone absolutely agreeing with Dr. Lewis's research.

I took the DHA throughout my entire deployment, and several times I was far too close to detonations. I sustained minor *fragmentation wounds when a grenade detonated approximately six to ten feet from me. Throughout my deployment and the countless times I was closer than we should have been to detonations, I never suffered any signs of TBI. I also know that I have depression despite that I have never been diagnosed because I just don't tell my health-care providers about the symptoms. During my nine-month deployment to Afghanistan I never once had an episode of depression. I attribute this absolutely to following the guidelines found in Dr. Lewis's research.*

After my deployment, I stopped taking the supplements because I was no longer exposed to the effects of explosives at all, if ever. I have not had any symptoms of TBI since I have been back, but I have definitely had bouts of depression. I have decided that I will begin taking the omega-3 supplements again because I felt healthier overall while taking them during my deployment.

While resiliency may come from genetics and I can't prove that my lack of TBI was absolutely from taking omega-3 supplements, I feel strongly that it was the omega-3 supplements that had a big part to do with me not getting TBI and certainly not suffering from depression. I hope that more people will pay attention to this research because I do believe that it will help my brothers in arms who have suffered TBI from over a decade of war.

Thank you.
Elijah

Elijah survived the IED explosions and remained in relatively good mental health, keeping depression at bay, because his brain was in balance. His consumption of fish oil prior to accidents protected his brain and kept it from a chronic, inflammatory state. His brain health, as measured by the ratio of omega-3s to omega-6s, was optimal, and his brain was able to withstand both physical and mental pressure.

PREVENTIVE NUTRITION

Starting in June 2014, Texas Christian University (TCU) began a concussion and nutrition study with their football team, the Horned Frogs. They enrolled their entire football team, all eighty-one players, in a randomized, double blind, placebo controlled study, and looked at using 0, 2, 4, or 6 grams, or 6,000 milligrams of algael oil omega-3s per day generously supplied by Martek-DSM, the NASA spin-off company I mentioned in chapter 3.

When the study was completed, they published their research as a medical journal article: "Effective Dose of Docosahexaenoic Acid on Biomarkers of Head Trauma in American Football." I did a bit of consulting with Jonathan Oliver, the lead investigator, when he was getting the study up and running. Graciously, Jonathan thanked me in the acknowledgment section, and I believe the study is incredibly important.

The study's duration was 189 days, from June 1 to

December 31, during the practice and football season. This was 2014, the year the Horned Frogs suffered just one loss and ended the year ranked third in the country. The TCU study was the first large-scale effort to (1) examine the potential prophylactic use of omega-3s in American football, and (2) identify the optimal dose of DHA to suggest a neuroprotective effect with supplementation. Additionally, they did a second study comparing baseline, pre-season blood measures of a possible biological marker of head trauma, and evaluated levels in players throughout the season. Published in the *Journal of Neurotrauma*, the TCU research team found substantial increases over the course of a football season of serum neurofilament light polypeptide protein, particularly in starting players. As they reported, "These data suggest that a season of collegiate American football is associated with elevations in serum NFL [neuro-filament light], which is indicative of axonal injury, as a result of head impacts."

The results of the DHA were equally impressive. After reviewing past concussion rates and rates of concussions on teams of similar size, investigators expected, on average, fourteen concussions that year. Yet, only six concussions were documented in the 2014 season. We don't know if it was because of the omega-3s or not, but a 50 percent drop in a single year is compelling even though the numbers are too small to really put a lot of scientific credence into it. More importantly, they found that DHA attenuated or decreased the amount of serum neurofilament light. Basically, supplementation with DHA reduced this important biomarker associated with head injury.

This study, published in the journal *Medicine & Science in Sports & Exercise*, makes clear that while American football athletes are exposed to subconcussive impacts over the course of a season resulting in elevations of biomarkers of axonal injury, taking omega-3s is imperative to help protect the brain from impacts. DHA clearly decreased the amount of this head trauma biomarker in these athletes. Who knows? Maybe DHA even helped TCU to have a better season and finish number 3 in the final poll!

On a serendipitous note, before TCU began their study, the lead investigator at TCU contacted me. He wanted advice about how to structure the study. Realistically, the concussion rate for the football team was not going to be zero and he wanted to plan with their sports medicine doctor, saying, "We're in the process of putting this study together, knowing injuries will occur. We're trying to figure out what do we do with the players that do suffer a head injury."

We all got on the phone, and the sports-medicine trained team physician spoke up and explained, "I already used omega-3s in my concussion patients." She then described, word for word, The Omega-3 Protocol. "I start them off on fifteen capsules a day for at least a week and then I decrease it ten capsules a day or two doses for the second week and get them down to one dose a day the week after."

I couldn't help myself. "Does it work?"

"Yes, every time. It works great."

I was curious. "Where did you hear about that?"

"I heard about it from a scientific conference."

"That's my protocol!"

She wasn't really sure how the information reached her, but she was using The Omega Protocol because she had investigated its merits and decided to try it with concussed football players. The next step was her quest to see if omega-3s could be taken as a supplement and shore up the brain to protect it from concussion. As the results proved, the answer is yes.

HOW ARE OMEGA-3S PRODUCED?

In November 2013, I received an email from a man whose introduction was both intriguing and personal. The email opened with, "I wanted to reach out to you because of the work you're doing with omega-3s for TBI. I've read your research, saw your Omega-3 Protocol for brain injury, and it made me think that this protocol should be applied to athletes in contact sports to help the brain recover from hits they take on the field. In college I played for the University of Chicago."

It turned out he was a captain of the University of Chicago football team and then started playing rugby for the Chicago Lions, one of the better rugby clubs in the United States. He and another rugby teammate, an all-American rugby player at the University of Minnesota, asked me for advice. They wanted to start a business focused on athletes and health and decided they wanted to make an omega-3 fish oil product that would make following The Omega-3 Protocol easier than taking a hand full of capsules. Rather than playing with capsules, they decided they were going to put all the omega-3s in a two-ounce bottle, like a five-hour energy drink. Using their own funding, they launched their idea in a bottle. Today, they sell Re:Mind Recover with 3,000 milligrams of EPA and DHA in a single, shot-glass-sized bottle, to drink. They are marketing specifically to athletes looking for protection from head injury.

These two men from Chicago were hungry, aggressive, and young. They wanted to start a business and target athletes. As part of their marketing study, they started calling college athletic departments and making those personal connections. What they found was surprising. More than half of the athletic departments of colleges around the country were already using or recommending omega-3s for the prevention of head injury or after to help recovery from concussions. Yet, no one is talking about this. And this silence has spread to the NFL. Several NFL teams have quietly made fish oil available to their athletes, but, publicly they won't admit to offering nutritive support. My hope is that with more than half of the athletic departments in the country using fish oil, the other half will follow.

WHAT OTHER CONDITIONS CAN OMEGA-3S HELP WITH?

As pointed out before, other conditions benefit from fish oil. This data comes partly from the experience through the nonprofit and emails from people who self-select to contact me. But there is also strong support in the scientific literature, including omega-3s' positive behavioral effect on patients with ADHD, autism, anxiety, and depression—just to name a few mental-health challenges.

In November 2012, I received an email from a representative with the New York City Metro chapter of National Autism Association. She wrote:

"I've been following your research and have started my nine-year-old, autistic son with your protocol of high dose omega-3s. It's well documented that children with autism have neuroinflammation, idling neurons, and altered immune functioning, so it was a natural fit to try this protocol with my son. The results we are seeing in attention, language, eye contact, and cognition are incredible, and all within the first week of starting the protocol."

Another woman wrote about her autistic grandson and revealed, "It's been two weeks since my grandson began the high-dose omega-3s you recommend, and we continue to see amazing results. My grandson is so much more present. His eye contact has never been better. His cognition continues to grow every day, and his therapists are all commenting on how fast he is mastering his program. His occupational therapist is also seeing great results in writing and cutting skills, not to mention gross motor skills. Every day is so exciting because we can't wait to see what he will be able to accomplish." Children diagnosed with autism can also present rage cycles, where they are overwhelmed by stimuli or their own emotions, which they don't understand, and they cannot stay in control. What I have found is that omega-3s decrease the frequency and intensity of these rage cycles.

In terms of children with ADHD, there are many studies that point to the efficacy of using fish oil in behavioral treatment plans. Just in March 2015, a study demonstrated that boys diagnosed with ADHD may benefit from omega-3 supplements. At the end of the study, boys who consumed the omega-3 supplements saw a reduction in their attention problems, as rated by their parents. Improvements in increasing attention spans were also documented. Another important 2011 study by the National Center for Biotechnology Information (NCBI), concluded "Omega-3 fatty acid supplementation, particularly with higher doses of Eicosapentaenoic acids, was modestly effective in the treatment of ADHD." The NCBI went on to add that the omega-3 fatty acid supplementation produced "modest" gains compared with currently available pharmacological interventions, and "given its relatively benign side-effect profile and evidence of modest efficacy, it might be reasonable to use omega-3 fatty supplementation to augment tradition pharmacologic interventions." They added, "Increased levels of omega-3s are associated with improved literacy, attention, and behavior."

There are over 150 scientific studies, in both the United States and abroad, focusing on omega-3s and their impact on individuals with ADHD that echo these conclusions.

Recently, the New York Times published a story on omega-3s and decreased violence. Happily titled "Does Eating Salmon Lower the Murder Rate?" by Steven Mihm, the article highlights studies that describe how consuming more omega-3s tends to lower the level of violence and rage among adults, particularly those incarcerated. This article supports the findings of my buddy, Joe Hibbeln, who published his study with the NIH under the equally provocative title, "Sea Food Consumption and Homicide Mortality." Joe found a direct correlation between a higher intake of omega-3 fatty acids and lower murder rates.

In 2002, Dr. Bernard Finch designed a placebo-controlled, double-blinded, randomized trial looking at 231 prisoners and assigned half of them to the nutritional intervention with omega-3s and half of them to a placebo. What they found was that those receiving the omega-3s had 37% fewer serious offenses involving violence and

26% fewer offenses overall. Moral of the story? An omega-3 fed brain is a calmer brain.

SOURCES OF OMEGA-3

The best sources of omega-3s are deep, cold-water fish, including Arctic cod, anchovies, flounder, mackerel, salmon, and squid. The American Heart Association recommends eating a variety of fish, preferably oily fish—for example, salmon, tuna, or herring—up to six ounces a week or two three-ounce servings of fish per week. The levels of omega-3s will differ with the fish and the source of the fish, but fish sticks and tilapia are not adequate sources of omega-3s. On the other hand, a mere three ounces of herring, salmon, or mackerel will provide more than 1500 milligrams of omega-3s.

Another benefit of actually consuming real fish is what is called the "whole food effect." This means you are not only receiving the benefits of the proteins and omega-3s, but you are also reaping benefits from what are known as "micro-nutrients." With salmon, in particular, you get a dose of a micronutrient called astaxanithin. This is the substance that gives salmon its rich pink color.

Astaxanithin is a carotenoid, a really powerful anti-oxidant, and it is from the same chemical soup that makes carrots orange...thus the reason we call them "carrots" (from the word *carotenoid*). The amount of astaxanithin is important, and the rule of thumb is the more the better.

This demonstrates the issue of farmed fish versus wild-caught salmon. Again, the food supply should remain as pristine as possible because you are what you eat. Farmed fish, however, are not so pristine. Farmed fish are fed limited foods themselves, which means their flesh and oils simply will not be as nutrient-rich as wild-caught fish.

If you go to the store and you look at the difference in the color between farmed salmon and wild-caught salmon, you will see one of two things. In the farmed fish either the salmon flesh is very pale, with little astaxanthin, or it will be bright pink with food coloring, added just to make the salmon look healthy. The difference between farmed and wild salmon, or any fish, is that the wild fish are rich in micronutrients as they accumulate in the food chain. You don't get a rich food-chain effect from farmed fish. That's why there's such a big difference between the two and why eating wild fish is so much better for you.

Whenever I give talks about fish oil or eating fish, I am approached by parents and spouses concerned with eating wild fish or taking fish oil and the potential exposure to mercury. This is more of a pressing concern in pregnant women. Years ago, the US government came out with a warning that pregnant women should avoid all fish. This ruling is now considered outdated and is about to be scrapped by the NIH. What happened was that the recommendations advising pregnant women to avoid eating fish were based completely on the EPA's recommendation to avoid mercury, and there was no input from the NIH or the FDA on the recommended amounts of omega-3s pregnant women should consume.

What has since been determined is the potential exposure to mercury from eating the recommended two portions of fish per week is actually negligible. A pregnant woman can also just eat fish known to have lower mercury levels. In terms of IQ points, what they've calculated out now is that potential exposure to mercury equates to a loss of one half of an IQ point in the child. However, the lack of omega-3s, by not eating fish during pregnancy, correlates to a loss of seven IQ points in the child. By not eating fish, you lose the potential for gaining seven IQ points by trying to avoid a potential loss of half an IQ point.

In short, as far as mercury levels in fish are concerned, the higher on the food chain, the larger the fish, and the more concentrated the pollutants. This is a concept called bioaccumulation. If the little fish have a little bit of mercury, and the next-sized fish eats them, and so forth, all that mercury accumulates as you go up the food chain. The bigger fish, such as Chilean sea bass, marlin, grouper, swordfish, shark, and some tuna are known to have the highest levels of mercury. The good news is that salmon, anchovies, mackerel, and trout tend to have the lowest. The rule of thumb is to use common sense. We know canned tuna tends to actually be fairly high in mercury, so avoid it.

For vegetarians and vegans, there are omega-3s sourced from oil extracted from algae grown in million-gallon tanks. Here the oil is extracted directly from the algae. Remember those NASA scientists who started Martek-DSM? Their product is certified is for vegans and Halal, and it is an ideal vegetarian alternative to fish oil made from micro-algae, which offers a plant-based source of beneficial marine omega-3 EPA and DHA without the use of fish. Certified by the American Vegetarian Association, it is also non-GMO.

While shopping for fish oil, you may also run across omega-3s sourced from krill. Krill are tiny sea animals, near the start of the seafood chain, and processing krill oil for mass consumption is relatively new. Krill oil tends to be very expensive compared to fish oil and has much lower levels of omega-3s. Though pushed hard right now in the marketplace, krill oil is inferior to fish and fish oil capsules. Krill oil may have a slightly higher percentage of phospholipids than fish oil, but all marine-sourced oils have a percentage of phospholipids and a percentage of triglycerides. Dollar for dollar, you get a lot more omega-3s from fish oil than you do from krill oil.

WHAT TO LOOK FOR ON THE LABEL

Reading fish oil labels is tricky. Google "how to read a fish oil label," and you'll find there are 615,000 results. If you wander down the supplements isle of your grocery store, you will see many varieties of fish oil, from orangey capsules to clear yellow ones announcing how "odorless" they are on the label. It gets confusing fast. What you are looking for is a basic fish oil or salmon oil.

When you're going to buy fish oil, pull out a bottle and check the label. Learn how to read fish oil labels and learn to look for important information, which includes the source, serving size, and the ingredients. First, you want to look at the source for where the fish come from: anchovies, sardines, or salmon. These tend to be the most commonly used sources of fish oil and the most plentiful.

Second, you want to look at the serving size, so that you can add up how many capsules to take to create The Omega-3 Protocol either for a daily maintenance dose or for concussion or for severe TBI. The critical piece of information is how many milligrams of EPA and DHA are in a single capsule or serving.

Many capsules are described by "serving," and a serving may be two capsules, so don't forget to divide by two to determine how much EPA and DHA are in an individual capsule. The combined EPA and DHA percentages should be about 50 to 60 percent of the amount of the entire capsule. For example, if it is a 1,000 milligram capsule, there should be at least 500 milligrams of EPA and DHA. Even better would be 600 milligrams.

Third, you should check the ingredients. The source is the fish, but the ingredients are what the capsules or the oil is emulsified and processed with. Though soy is often listed, there's so little that it does not matter. More critical is the grade of oil. Ideally your fish oil should be pharmaceutical grade, molecularly distilled, and in a triglyceride form that meets or surpasses the strictest international standards for purity and freshness. They should be able to provide you with a certificate of analysis if you request it.

All fish oil keeps better in a cool, dark place, but most capsules or liquid fish oil come in either dark glass or plastic containers that protect the contents from light.

WHAT TO WATCH FOR AND AVOID

There are, however, some ingredients, by-products, and sources to avoid. You want to find a fish oil supplement where the oil is extracted as triglycerides versus ethyl esters. Basically, if you squeeze a fish, you get triglycerides. This is the molecular form that makes up virtually all fats and oils in plants and animals. The omega-3 fatty acids naturally found in fish are almost exclusively triglycerides.

Triglycerides are three molecules on a glycerol backbone. What happens in molecular distillation is the glycerol backbone is chemically broken in order to free up those three fatty acids. The fatty acids are essentially molecularly distilled by attaching them to an ethanol molecule. An "ethyl ester" is one fatty-acid chain attached to one ethanol molecule. Ethyl esters are not found in nature but are created through chemical synthesis. Technically, they're not even an oil.

This molecular distillation not only separates out the fatty-acid chain ethyl esters but also releases toxins, mercury, and heavy metals that can be scrubbed and removed. When the ethyl ester is molecularly distilled and cleaned, it can then be converted back into the triglyceride form. This is called re-esterification. This means a company can re-esterfy the fatty acids back to the triglyceride bone, and re-create the triglyceride oil. As you can imagine, this is a much more natural form that can be easily digested and metabolized. This process is costly, however, and often bypassed by many fish oil manufacturers, including those producing pharmaceutical fish oils requiring a prescription.

The result is that most fish oil capsules are actually in ethyl ester form and therefore are not even technically a fish oil. Most capsules of fish oil are ethyl esters and most liquid forms are triglycerides. Liquid ethyl ester products are rare because they degrade faster, spoil quicker, and carry a much more intense fishy flavor, making them less palatable. Because ethyl esters are not found in nature, our digestive systems don't know how to digest the ethyl ester very efficiently. They are very poorly absorbed compared to the triglycerides found in nature and in seafood. Ethyl esters also tend to "repeat" on the consumer. This means you may have indigestion and erupt with a very unpleasant, fishy burp.

According to a good friend of mine, Carlos Montesinos, the formulation scientist who designs all nutritional products and nutritional supplement products for the NASA space program, if a fish oil "repeats" on you, it was either poorly manufactured or the product has spoiled. A good fish oil should never repeat. You should remain burp-free. If the burp test seems a bit flimsy and you cannot tell from the label if the oil was converted back to triglycerides, then check with the manufacturer.

PEOPLE WILL NOTICE A DIFFERENCE BETWEEN A GOOD AND NOT-SO-GOOD PRODUCT

A few years ago, I got this nice email that really drives the point home:

"I forgot to tell you about my eighteen-year-old autistic grandson. We switched him to the less expensive omega-3. His mom told him there was no difference and he would have the same improvements as the Nordic Naturals fish oil. Clarity of mind, more upbeat. Approximately one week after the change, he went to his mom and said, 'I know you said I wouldn't notice a difference, but I do. I don't think my thinking is as clear and I don't think my mood is as upbeat.' So expecting no change, he still noticed a change. He convinced me and his mom there is a difference and again the cost is well worth it."

My sixteen-year-old son plays high school football and lacrosse. People often ask me, "How can you let your son play such violent sports? Aren't you worried about him getting a concussion?" Of course I'm concerned, but I value team sports such as football and lacrosse so much that the benefits outweigh the risk. But there are things we can do to mitigate the risks as I mentioned before. So my son, as well as the rest of my family including myself, doesn't leave the breakfast table every single day of the year without taking 3,000 milligrams of EPA/DHA—five capsules every single morning.

NO SUBSTITUTE FOR EATING HEALTHY—TED WADE'S ORDEAL

Ted Wade was a soldier in the 82nd Airborne. Ted didn't find the Army rations that arrived in packets, succulently titled MREs or "meals ready to eat," a culinary delight. To put it less eloquently, Ted didn't like Army grub. He also knew he needed more nutritional food.

In response to Ted's plea for better food, his fiancée, Sarah, sent him jars of fish oil capsules, salmon jerky, canned tuna, canned salmon, and sardines. When he would go out on patrols, he would make his own meals from the omega-3 rich foods Sarah sent him. He ate very, very differently than most people in the Army, and he felt better knowing he was better off eating seafood. Unlike most of his fellow soldiers with low omega-3 intake, his omega-3 intake was high. Ultimately, it was the omega-3s that helped save his life.

In February 2004, Ted's Humvee struck an IED on a mission in Al-Mahmudiyah, Iraq, and the vehicle exploded. He suffered a traumatic amputation of his right arm, multiple fractured bones, soft-tissue shrapnel injuries, and complications due to a number of other injuries. Though in a coma, the Army medevaced Ted to a military medical facility in Germany. No one expected him to survive. His condition was so critical that the Army wasn't comfortable authorizing further travel back to Walter Reed for care. His doctors did not think he would survive the flight across the Atlantic so he was transferred from the US Army hospital to a local German hospital that dealt with severe injuries. Ted's father and Sarah were contacted and encouraged to fly to Germany and say their good-byes. Sarah and Ted's father immediately flew to Germany, to the hospital's ICU, hoping he'd still be alive. He was. Ted held his own in a coma for more than two months when the recommendation came that his father should make a decision to end life support. But his father never had to make that decision because Ted woke from his coma.

The medical protocol around the treatment of TBI in Germany is different than it is in the states. In Germany, real food is routinely ground up and put down a feeding tube. Here, in the United States, we tend to rely on Carnation instant breakfast and canned liquid protein drinks. But in Germany, Ted's doctors and nursing staff ground up fish, sardines, and vegetables, and fed him this real food, high in omega-3s. The staff would talk to him and stimulate his brain even though he was in a coma. Just as the question about life support came up, Ted began to stir.

When he came home, he and Sarah married. Ted has been able to heal and lead a normal life. Both Sarah and Ted believe his recovery from injuries deemed fatal is the result of having a prepared brain: all that tuna, salmon, and the fish oil supplements saved his life. Rather than being out of balance with too many omega-6s, Ted's brain was already reaping the benefits of a brain fed with omega-3s.

CONCLUSION

FRIENDLY NEIGHBORS

Sometimes the preventive or beneficial effects of fish oil are a complete surprise to all concerned parties. Where we used to live, my next neighbor was an official at a foreign embassy in Washington, DC. One day, he was goofing around and decided to climb a large tree in the middle of my backyard. He fell, broke his collar bone, sustained a traumatic brain injury, and was transported to the hospital. All this unfolded the day before I left to go overseas to Kyrgyzstan. My mission was for a week.

I felt terrible, of course, about the accident. Before I left, I gave his wife a bottle of algae-sourced fish oil, certified for vegans. In the past, we had inspired conversations over nutrition, and I knew he, his wife, and three children were strict kosher vegans. I told her about The

Omega Protocol and gave her the instructions and how much her husband should take.

After my return seven days later, I popped over next door and asked how her husband was feeling. "Oh, he's doing much better," she said serenely.

"Did he notice a difference by taking the omega-3 oil?"

"What do you mean?" Then she looked confused. "I took the omega-3 oil. I thought you brought that for me."

She assumed as the mother of three young, robust boys, I had offered omega-3 oil to help her through her days of single parenting while her husband recuperated.

"Well, I took it and I feel great. I've never been calmer, or more relaxed. I never realized I could be this calm and relaxed with three young boys running around the house."

Her brain needed nutritional support while her husband's brain healed. She bought a second bottle for him.

FINAL THOUGHTS

Concussions and TBI, with their diverse heterogeneity and prolonged secondary pathogenesis, remains a clinical challenge for the medical community. Clinical studies thus far continue to fail to identify an effective pharmaceutical strategy when a combination of targets controlling aspects of neuroprotection, neuroinflammation, and neuroregeneration is needed. Omega-3s offer the advantage of this combination approach.

There is a growing body of strong pre-clinical evidence

and clinical experience suggesting that benefits are possible from aggressively adding substantial amounts of omega-3s to optimize the nutritional foundation of TBI, concussion, and postconcussive syndrome patients. Even early and optimal doses of omega-3s, in a prophylactic setting, have the potential to improve outcomes from this devastating problem.

With evidence of unsurpassed safety and tolerability, omega-3s should be considered mainstream, conventional medicine. Conventional medicine must overcome its inherent bias against nutritional, nonpharmacologic therapies. One of my biggest frustrations as a physician trying to change one approach to how TBI and concussion medicine is practiced is how closed-minded other physicians can be at times.

How do we overcome medicine's inherent bias? That challenge is up to all of us as concerned patients, parents, and physicians.

WHATEVER HAPPENED TO BOBBY?

As you've seen, patients suffering from a variety of problems, not just traumatic brain injuries and concussions, can often be helped with an increase or introduction to fish oil. But there is another oil rich in omega-3s that can specifically be used in patients with depression and anxiety: hemp-derived CBD oil.

CBD oil, or cannabidiol oil, is derived from hemp,

one of the two cannabis sativa plants, the other being marijuana. Although they are lumped together phylogenetically, marijuana and hemp are very different. What's interesting to note is that while marijuana has been deemed by the FDA as a Schedule 1 Drug and is highly controlled, the NIH holds a patent on the medical use of CBD, cannabidiol. The name of the patent is "Cannabidiol as a Neuro-protectant and Antioxidant." One of the authors of that patent is a Nobel Prize researcher who first described serotonin in neurotransmitters. CBD not only helps protect the brain from injury, but is highly effective treating cases of depression and anxiety and it's available as a nutritional supplement.

The story of Bobby continues here, at this point. Four years after his accident, Bobby was struggling with depression and anxiety in spite of the fish oil he continues to take. This is common with patients who have suffered a severe traumatic brain injury. When I learned about CBD, this hemp-derived oil, I contacted Bobby and his family to see if he would be willing to try it. The studies from the NIH were compelling, and I was able to convince Bobby to try CV Sciences +PlusCBD Gold derived from hemp. Two weeks after he began this new, augmented protocol, his father called me to report, "This is unbelievable. This has been a life-changing drug that you've got Bobby on."

But CBD is not a drug. It is simply nutritional support, full of omega-3s that stimulate and heal the brain. When

Bobby took the phone, his voice sounded light. "Dr. Lewis," he said, "thank you so much. This has really changed my life. I'm no longer depressed. I stopped taking my anti-depressants. I'm not feeling depressed in the least bit. I feel better than I have since the accident." He continued, "And my anxiety levels have come down so much so that I actually asked a girl for her phone number. I never would have done that before."

Bobby noticed an improvement within two weeks of starting to take the +PlusCBD Gold oil. I've suggested this protocol with just a handful of patients. I've also treated a thirteen-year-old-girl whom I've been working with for three years. CBD has kept her anxiety levels the lowest they've ever been since her brain injury. In all cases, the brain is calmed and able to function at its best. Neither omega-3s nor CBD are a cure for TBI, ADHD, autism, or anxiety, but by feeding the brain what it needs to function well, they prepare each brain to function as best it can.

If ever there is a doubt that I'm making a difference in peoples' lives, this email from Bobby certainly can change that:

Dr. Lewis,

Thank you so much for giving me CBD oil. It drastically changed my life, I cannot begin to describe it with words. Thanks to CBD oil, I'm feeling much more comfortable in my own skin, I'm being more social, and I'm making BIG noticeable changes. I'm doing stand-up comedy now, I have my own place, I got a raise at my job, and I'm feeling VERY optimistic about the future! A friend I made when I was doing improv comedy told me, and I've also been told repeatedly this, that I have a great personality and a great ZEST for life! You gave my life back again. I can't wait to see what adventures come next in life.

RESOURCES

THE BRAIN HEALTH EDUCATION AND RESEARCH INSTITUTE

While traveling and speaking around the country, I am often asked, "Why start a nonprofit?" The answer lies in my lifetime experience in both service and science.

Retirement is not really a word that resonates with me. However, after a productive and rewarding thirty-one-and-a-half-year career in the US Army, I felt ready for the next step, and another challenge in my professional life. I also knew I was sitting on information that would help those who suffered concussion or severe TBI and I wanted to reach out to patients and their families as well as their doctors. I found the research exciting and working with patients rewarding. Clearly, I needed to find a way to reach a broader and more diverse audience, and educate families, moms and dads, both military and civilian. The new information and research about how omega-3s can help heal traumatic brain injury and concussion were so compelling that I wanted to develop a center where information could be consolidated.

About once a month, I would meet up with a good friend for breakfast. Month after month, he would encourage me to set up a website and make my protocols available to the world. I just couldn't see the business model. He would talk about gaining viewership and selling advertising space, but I'm just not a natural salesman. Then one day he said something like, "You know everyone in the field. Why don't you create a board of advisors for your website I've been telling you to start?" Given my training and board certification in preventive medicine and public health, it finally made sense to me. I didn't need a website to get this information out to people. I needed a nonprofit with a website to disseminate this information to people. The Brain Health Education and Research Institute is the result of hard work and a pressing need to seek discovery. I have chosen to take a public health approach with my nonprofit and reach that larger audience. Change happens incrementally and in leaps, and my hope is BHERI manages both.

BHERI's purpose is twofold. One goal is to change how the medical community practices the treatment of, and interventions for, concussion and traumatic brain injury. This change focuses on educating the medical community on the importance of nutritional support and the critical necessity of supplementation with omega-3s. Our second goal is to establish and grow a grassroots approach of reaching the community of concerned patients and parents, and to help educate them about what they can do to improve brain health both preventively and after injury occurs. I want to reach what I call the three Ps: the patients, the parents, and the providers of health care. BHERI is uniquely situated to reach all three with information about nutritional support and The Omega Protocol, to offer resources for families, and to disseminate compelling studies and new developments in treatment for TBI.

The Brain Health Education and Research Institute's mission is to change the way we address protection from, and treatment of, all forms brain injury. From proactively taking care of our brain health on an ongoing basis, to post injury treatment, to recovery, BHERI is committed to being at the forefront of research and education. BHERI supports continuing research on omega-3s (ALA, DHA, and EPA) and their impact on brain health. By designing and directing research as well as reviewing the latest research from NIH and major universities, BHERI is providing solutions to brain health issues.

There are real, proactive benefits of omega-3s in the diet to improve lives and protect people from the long-term implications of brain injury. Ultimately, BHERI provides comprehensive educational resources and tools about how to effectively facilitate recovery from brain injury through the use of omega-3 fatty acids.

Concerned parents, patients, or providers searching for answers and solutions to concussions, TBI, and other head injury beyond the traditional and largely outdated recommendations can come to BHERI's website and learn about the newest solutions for the most effective recovery possible.

One of BHERI's greatest interests is protecting children. Nourishing a child's brain is incredibly important to his or her future health and happiness. Early nutritional support sets the stage for ongoing brain health and can help reduce the risks of disease, dementia, as well as the ability to recover from common injuries like concussions.

But BHERI's main research objective remains the same: to develop, guide, fund, and oversee critical research necessary to cultivate the scientific foundation to answer clinical questions about the use of omega-3s for a variety of conditions including concussions, PTSD, and other psychological conditions. The NIH and other sources fund basic studies in this area; however, true clinical research efforts are few and disjointed. There are only a select number of omega-3 researchers in the field, and they are poorly funded and lack a unified direction. BHERI was founded to ask the right questions and guide the research, with an emphasis on clinical trials, to solve the difficult problems to benefit our soldiers, our children, and the sports community. In this way, our goal of reaching the three Ps—patients, parents, and providers of health care—is achievable.

For background information, I have many dozens of radio interviews and videos online. The Internet is a marvelous thing. Just search my name, "Dr. Michael Lewis and Omega-3s." You can search "Sanjay Gupta Lewis," "Bailes and Lewis," and an almost endless list of search words. All will yield interviews, videos, and published, peer-reviewed articles.

BHERI's website, brainhealtheducation.org, offers a wealth of information and sourced material. To stay abreast of recent developments in brain trauma and brain nutrition, regular updates, and the latest news and research on omega-3s and TBI, be sure to click on the box for our "Newsletter." Another box will take to "TBI and Concussion, Signs, Symptoms, and Help." A third offers information on "Advances in Head Injury Prevention and Management, What Else Can Be Done?" Podcasts, interviews, recent published papers and a link to my blog are all available.

If you find the information in this book or on the BHERI website, please consider two things:

1. Making a tax-free donation so we can reach out to more people and with enough donations, be able to fund research to answer more questions and change how medicine is practiced. Find us at www.brainhealtheducation.org/donate-to-the-institute

2. Sign up for the weekly BHERI newsletter that gives you the latest news and information about TBI, concussions, and nutrition interventions for brain health. Go to www.brain-healtheducation.org/newsletter/

A NEW CLINICAL PRACTICE CALLED BRAINCARE

Besides establishing BHERI, I recently decided to return to clinical care. People email me all the time asking me if they can come see me and where is my clinical practice. In the Army, you routinely change jobs every three to four years. I have been retired from the Army now for four years, so it feels like it is time to change things up again, so I've started a private practice called Brain-CARE (Concussion*Assessment*Recovery*Education). In this way, as a practicing doctor with a clinic devoted to TBI, concussions, and brain health, I can remain in close contact with patients and bring my experience and expertise in both diagnosing and treating brain injury to foster better brain health. I believe in an integrative medical approach that looks at the patient holistically and may assess a patient in different ways in addition to traditional medical examinations and lab tests. These assessments are useful in telling us how the brain is functioning, and in finding the root cause of health issues. We offer more treatment options and therapies for healing at the root cause of a head injury, not just treating the symptoms. As such, appointments are almost always longer than typical medical office visits, often lasting two or more hours. I believe in listening to the patient and the families. Often, there is much that can be learned about what the patient is really suffering just by listening. When is the last time your doctor's appointment lasted two hours?

At BrainCARE, I use progressive technologies and a comprehensive approach to optimize conditions to allow the injured brain to heal. Using a collaborative approach with referring physicians, my goal is to get patients back to optimal functioning. At BrainCARE, we'll work to help you with the following:

- Concussions
- Traumatic Brain Injury (TBI)
- ADD/ADHD
- Brain Fog
- Poor Concentration
- Sports Performance
- Concussion Prevention Strategies

Diagnosing a concussion is not always completely straight forward, especially if it happened weeks, months, or even years ago. We don't just rely on a computerized neurocognitive test. We use advanced diagnostics such as these:

- Detailed History and Physical
- Detailed Nutritional and Hormone Biomarker Evaluation

- Evoke Neuroscience Advanced EEG Brain Mapping
- Heart Rate Variability Evaluation
- Evoked Potential Brain Processing Speed Evaluation
- C3 Logix Concussion Evaluation
- Sway Diagnostics Balance Testing

I think the most important thing I can add as a health-care provider is approaching every patient as an individual and actually doing something. Telling a patient to go sit in a dark closet for two weeks is something you will never hear in my office. Instead we'll talk about actual therapies that can help patients get their lives back, such as the following:

- Targeted Nutritional Therapy
- Graduated Non-contact Exercise
- Bioidentical Hormone Replacement
- Near Infrared Light Therapy
- Heart Rate Variability Training
- 4-D sLORETA EEG Neurofeedback
- Nasal Release Technique

The brain is plastic, powerful, and able to heal. I am making it my mission in life to help patients reach their full healing potential and to assist their families in negotiating the best treatment plan for their loved ones. Correcting the imbalance that leaves us predisposed to concussion is one issue. Helping brains heal as best they can is the other. Part of the answer is in omega-3s.

This model, of establishing both a nonprofit and a medical practice, offers two avenues to reach the public and health-care professionals. BHERI stands as an educational think tank while BrainCARE offers actual clinical services. The combination of both organizations means I can help make an impact on how patients are treated and help patients heal as much, and as well, as they can.

Here are the best ways to reach me:

The address for both Brain Health Education and Research and the BrainCARE Clinic is 7811 Montrose Road, Suite 215, Potomac, Maryland 20854. Feel free to call the office at (240) 398-3481 to schedule an appointment or telephone consult. Or email to appointments@potomacbraincare.com.

Websites and Facebook pages:

BrainCARE.center or PotomacBrainCARE.com

www.facebook.com/PotomacBrainCARE/

www.brainhealtheducation.org

www.facebook.com/BrainHealthEducation/

RESOURCES FOR ATHLETES, PARENTS, COACHES, AND PHYSICIANS

Government websites for more information on concussions and brain injury:

- www.cdc.gov/traumaticbraininjury/
- www.cdc.gov/headsup/

- www.nlm.nih.gov/medlineplus/traumaticbraininjury.htm
- www.nlm.nih.gov/medlineplus/concussion.html
- www.ninds.nih.gov/disorders/tbi/tbi.htm

Nongovernment websites for more information on TBI, concussions, or omega-3s:

- www.brainhealtheducation.org
- www.webmd.com/brain/tc/traumatic-brain-injury-concussion-overview
- Numerous university and medical school websites
- GOED: Global Organization for EPA and DHA Omega-3s
- www.goedomega3.com (Note: GOED is a 501(c)(6) not-for-profit trade association committed to transparency and proper governance.)

Though these are manufacturers' websites, they are also excellent sources for general information:

- www.ascentahealth.com/omega-3-and-you/
- www.nordicnaturals.com/en/General_Public/Why_Omega-3s/542
- www.omega-research.com

How to check your blood levels for omega-3s and omega-6s with a fatty-acid analysis:

- Lipid Technologies at www.lipidlab.com
- www.omegaquant.com
- www.questdiagnostics.com/testcenter/testguide.action?dc=TS_Omega_3_6

One of the most common questions I am asked is "What brand of fish oil do you recommend?" There are hundreds, if not thousands, of brands of omega-3s and fish oil on the market including a few pharmaceutical prescription brands (I don't recommend these as they are typically in ethyl ester form). I have worked with the following companies in one way or another over the years or am at least familiar enough with their products that I can say to look at these for starters:

NORDIC NATURALS

www.nordicnaturals.com

Note: I have been working with Nordic Naturals as a consultant since I retired from the Army. It was their UltimateOmega liquid product that first introduced me to the power of omegas when it was used with Bobby. Their UltimateOmega retail line and ProOmega professional line of products are what I like to use, and the exact same oil is used in liquid and capsule forms. They now have an even more concentrated product called UltimateOmega-2X or ProOmega-2000 that provides 1000mg of combined EPA+DHA per softgel decreasing the number of softgels per dose to three. For liquids, the new UltimateOmega Xtra and ProOmega-D Xtra liquids provide 3,000 milligrams of combined EPA+DHA in 1 teaspoon (5 ml). You can order online at www.nordicnaturals.com/en/NNPF/ Register_as_a_Patient/842, and use my provider #39160 for a 15% discount and free shipping.

PURE ENCAPSULATIONS

www.pureencapsulations.com

Note: Pure's O.N.E. Omega softgels provide 1000mg of EPA+DHA in triglyceride form, therefore requires only three softgels per dose. Additionally, Pure Encapsulations is my go-to product line for additional brain-healthy products such as: Cognitive Aminos, B-Complex w/ PQQ, Magnesium Citrate (for sleep), and O.N.E. Multivitamin. Order online at https://www.purecapspro.com/braincare/pe/home.asp for a discount.

DSM-MARTEK

www.lifesdha.com

Note: I almost became the Chief Medical Officer of Martek Biosciences before they were bought by DSM. Life's DHA products are derived from algae, not fish, and are certified as vegan, kosher, and halal. This product is perfect for vegetarians and is used in over 99 percent of infant formulas in the United States.

RE:MIND RECOVER

www.remindrecover.com

Note: A liquid form developed by two Chicago rugby players to make following The Omega-3 Protocol easier, Re:Mind Recover comes in 2-ounce bottles with a full dose of 3,000 milligrams combined EPA and DHA per bottle. I am on their Board of Advisors and helped guide

the development of this product. Order online at: https://
remindrecover.com/collections/all?rfsn=105149.2b9f22
for a discount.

AMERISCIENCES PRODUCTS BY NUGEVITY

www.amerisciences.com
Note: A company owned by my good friend and NASA
formulation specialist, Carlos Montesinos. These are
some of the highest-quality nutritional supplements
available. Under the auspice of a Space Act Agreement,
AmeriSciences products have been flown aboard both
Space Shuttle and International Space Station missions.
I particularly like their MM6 Multivitamin line and Ome-
gaMax line. I am on the Board of Advisors.

VITAL CHOICE WILD SEAFOOD & ORGANICS

www.vitalchoice.com
Note: Owned by good friend, Randy Hartnell, a twenty-
year veteran Alaskan fisherman, Vital Choice has the
absolute best-quality seafood available to ship direct. If
you want great salmon, here is the place, especially the
King Salmon. Their supplements are in triglyceride form
and sourced from Alaska.

WILEY'S FINEST

www.wileysfinest.com
Note: A family-owned and -run business in Ohio, Wiley's

products come from a responsible, sustainable, wild Alaskan fish source. Their liquid products are in triglyceride form.

COROMEGA

www.coromega.com

Note: Coromega products come in a flavored emulsion formula of triglycerides in squeeze packets (like a ketchup packet). They are great tasting and come in several different flavors. They're a great alternative for kids who won't swallow capsules or don't like liquid products.

ASCENTA

www.ascentahealth.com

Note: This is a Canadian company known for its high-quality NutraSea liquid products. They now have NutraVeg, an algae-based omega-3 supplement.

VAYA PHARMA

www.vayapharma.com

Note: This is an Israeli company that combines phosphatidylserine with either EPA (Vayarin) or DHA (Vayacog). Both products are marketed in the United States as medical foods, meaning they are only carried at pharmacies and your physician has to write a prescription.

CV SCIENCES HEMP-DERIVED CBD OIL

www.pluscbdoil.com

Note: While not technically an omega-3 product, cannabidiol (CBD) is a phytocannabinoid found in agricultural
hemp. I've found it is a helpful adjunct for anxiety and
stress relief and is also helpful in depression. I particularly like the plusCBDoil Gold 15mg softgels. I am on the
Board of Advisors.

These are not the only "good" brands out there, just the
ones with which I am most familiar. Remember that many
capsule products are not in the triglyceride form but the
much inferior ethyl ester form. Liquid products will almost
always be in triglyceride form because of the taste.

ABOUT THE AUTHOR

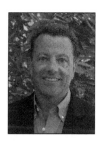 **MICHAEL D. LEWIS, MD, MPH, MBA, FACPM, FACN** is the president and founder of the Brain Health Education and Research Institute. He is an expert on nutritional and holistic interventions for brain health, particularly the use of omega-3 fatty acids for the prevention, management, and rehabilitation of concussions and traumatic brain injury (TBI). He founded the Brain Health Education and Research Institute in late 2011 upon retiring as a Colonel after a distinguished thirty-one-year career in the US Army.

His pioneering work in the military and since has helped thousands of people around the world and is regularly featured in the media, including CNN's Sanjay Gupta, MD, show and numerous radio shows and podcasts. He is a graduate of the US Military Academy at West Point and Tulane University School of Medicine. Dr. Lewis is board-certified and a fellow of the American Colleges of Preventive Medicine and Nutrition. He completed postgraduate training at Walter Reed Army Medical Center, Johns Hopkins University, and Walter Reed Army Institute of Research.

He is currently in private practice in Potomac, Maryland (BrainCARE, www.BrainCARE.center); is a consultant to the US Army and Navy as well as several organizations, institutes, and nutrition companies around the world; and is a founding member of the Pop Warner Youth Football Medical Advisory Board.

Printed in Great Britain
by Amazon